Precision Medicine in Practice: Molecular Diagnosis Enabling Precision Therapies

Editor

RYAN J. SCHMIDT

CLINICS IN LABORATORY MEDICINE

www.labmed.theclinics.com

Consulting Editor
MILENKO JOVAN TANASIJEVIC

June 2020 • Volume 40 • Number 2

ELSEVIER

1600 John F. Kennedy Boulevard • Suite 1800 • Philadelphia, Pennsylvania, 19103-2899

http://www.theclinics.com

CLINICS IN LABORATORY MEDICINE Volume 40, Number 2
June 2020 ISSN 0272-2712, ISBN-13: 978-0-323-75845-1

Editor: Katerina Heidhausen
Developmental Editor: Laura Fisher

Reprints. For copies of 100 or more, of articles in this publication, please contact the Commercial Reprints Department, Elsevier Inc., 360 Park Avenue South, New York, New York 10010-1710. Tel. 212-633-3874, Fax: 212-633-3820, E-mail: reprints@elsevier.com.

Clinics in Laboratory Medicine (ISSN 0272-2712) is published quarterly by Elsevier Inc., 360 Park Avenue South, New York, NY 10010-1710. Months of issue are March, June, September, and December. Business and Editorial offices: 1600 John F. Kennedy Blvd., Suite 1800, Philadelphia, PA 19103-2899. Periodicals postage paid at NewYork, NY and additional mailing offices. Subscription prices are $277.00 per year (US individuals), $571.00 per year (US institutions), $100.00 per year (US students), $349.00 per year (Canadian individuals), $693.00 per year (Canadian institutions), $100.00 per year (Canadian students), $404.00 per year (international individuals), $693.00 per year (international institutions), $185.00 (international students). Foreign air speed delivery is included in all Clinics subscription prices. All prices are subject to change without notice. POSTMASTER: Send address changes to *Clinics in Laboratory Medicine*, Elsevier Health Sciences Division, Subscription Customer Service, 3251 Riverport Lane, Maryland Heights, MO 63043. **Customer Service: 1-800-654-2452 (US). From outside of the US and Canada, call 1-314-447-8871. Fax: 1-314-447-8029. E-mail: journalscustomerservice-usa@elsevier.com (for print support) or journalsonlinesupport-usa@elsevier.com (for online support).**

Clinics in Laboratory Medicine is covered in *EMBASE/Exerpta Medica, MEDLINE/PubMed (Index Medicus), Cinahl, Current Contents/Clinical Medicine, BIOSIS* and *ISI/BIOMED.*

Contributors

EDITOR-IN-CHIEF

MILENKO JOVAN TANASIJEVIC, MD, MBA
Vice Chair for Clinical Pathology and Quality, Department of Pathology, Director of Clinical Laboratories, Brigham and Women's Hospital, Dana-Farber Cancer Institute, Associate Professor of Pathology, Harvard Medical School, Boston, Massachusetts, USA

EDITOR

RYAN J. SCHMIDT, MD, PhD
Assistant Director, Clinical Genomics Laboratory, Center for Personalized Medicine, Department of Pathology and Laboratory Medicine, Children's Hospital Los Angeles, Assistant Professor of Clinical Pathology, Keck School of Medicine of USC, Los Angeles, California, USA

AUTHORS

MARNI J. FALK, MD
Executive Director, CHOP Mitochondrial Medicine Frontier Program, Associate Professor, Division of Human Genetics, Department of Pediatrics, University of Pennsylvania Perelman School of Medicine, The Children's Hospital of Philadelphia, Philadelphia, Pennsylvania, USA

XIAOWU GAI, PhD
Associate Professor of Clinical Pathology, Keck School of Medicine of USC, Director of Bioinformatics, Center for Personalized Medicine, Children's Hospital Los Angeles, Los Angeles, California, USA

LIMIN HAO, PhD
Senior Bioinformatician, Bioinformatics and Laboratory of Molecular Medicine, Partners Personalized Medicine, Cambridge, Massachusetts, USA

ELAN HAHN, MD
Department of Laboratory Medicine and Pathobiology, University of Toronto, Toronto, Ontario, Canada

MATTHEW HIEMENZ, MD, MS
Department of Pathology and Laboratory Medicine, Children's Hospital Los Angeles, Department of Pathology, Keck School of Medicine of USC, Los Angeles, California, USA

NICOLE KOULISIS, MD
Department of Surgery, The Vision Center, The Saban Research Institute, Children's Hospital Los Angeles, USC Roski Eye Institute, Keck School of Medicine of USC, University of Southern California, Los Angeles, California, USA

MATTHEW S. LEBO, PhD, FACMG
Director, Bioinformatics and Laboratory of Molecular Medicine, Partners Personalized Medicine, Cambridge, Massachusetts, USA; Assistant Professor, Pathology, Harvard Medical School, Brigham and Women's Hospital, Boston, Massachusetts, USA

CHIAO-FENG LIN, PhD
Senior Bioinformatician, Bioinformatics and Laboratory of Molecular Medicine, Partners Personalized Medicine, Cambridge, Massachusetts, USA

ELIZABETH M. McCORMICK, MS, LCGC
Senior Genetic Counselor and Research Coordinator, Mitochondrial Medicine Frontier Program, Children's Hospital of Philadelphia, Philadelphia, Pennsylvania, USA

JESSICA MESTER, MS
Senior Genetic Counselor, GeneDx Inherited Cancer Program, Gaithersburg, Maryland, USA

COLLEEN CLARKE MURARESKU, MS, LCGC
Senior Genetic Counselor and Program Director, The Mitochondrial Medicine Frontier Program, The Children's Hospital of Philadelphia, Philadelphia, Pennsylvania, USA

DAVID R. MURDOCK, MD, FACMG
Assistant Professor, Department of Molecular and Human Genetics, Baylor College of Medicine, Houston, Texas, USA

AARON NAGIEL, MD, PhD
Department of Surgery, The Vision Center, The Saban Research Institute, Children's Hospital Los Angeles, USC Roski Eye Institute, Keck School of Medicine of USC, University of Southern California, Los Angeles, California, USA

RINI PAULY, MS
Greenwood Genetic Center, Greenwood, South Carolina, USA

TINA PESARAN, MS, MA
Director, Variant Assessment Program, Ambry Genetics, Aliso Viejo, California, USA

HOLGER PROKISCH, PhD
Institute of Human Genetics, Klinikum rechts der Isar, Technische Universität München, Ismaninger Munich, Germany; Institute of Human Genetics, Helmholtz Zentrum München, Ingolstaedter Neuherberg, Germany

CHARLES E. SCHWARTZ, PhD
Greenwood Genetic Center, Greenwood, South Carolina, USA

LISHUANG SHEN, PhD
Sr Bioinformatics Scientist, Center for Personalized Medicine, Children's Hospital Los Angeles, Los Angeles, California, USA

ARTI SINGH, MS
Bioinformatics Data Engineer, Bioinformatics and Laboratory of Molecular Medicine, Partners Personalized Medicine, Cambridge, Massachusetts, USA

SARAH L. STENTON, MBChB, MPhil
Institute of Human Genetics, Klinikum rechts der Isar, Technische Universität München, Ismaninger Munich, Germany; Institute of Human Genetics, Helmholtz Zentrum München, Ingolstaedter Neuherberg, Germany

Contents

> The diagnostic rate of comprehensive genomic sequencing remains only 25% to 30% due to the difficulty in interpreting variants of uncertain significance and noncoding mutations and in elucidating downstream effects of these and other genetic changes. Unlike DNA sequencing, RNA sequencing (RNAseq) reveals the functional consequence of genetic variation through the detection of abnormal gene expression levels, differences in gene splicing, and allele-specific expression. RNAseq can provide nearly 40% improvement in diagnostic rates depending on disease and tissue source. In this burgeoning era of precision medicine, RNAseq offers a powerful tool to improve diagnostic rates and understand disease mechanisms.

> Molecular genetic approaches have evolved at an astonishing pace resulting in increasingly routine use of whole exome sequencing in Mendelian disorder diagnosis. After whole exome sequencing, 50% to 75% of patients remain without a genetic diagnosis, indicating limitations in variant calling and prioritization and a role for noncoding variants. Whole genome sequencing has the potential to reveal all genetic variants; however, it escalates the challenge of variant prioritization owing to the vast numbers called. Promising approaches to aid in variant interpretation include the integration of functional genomic data such as transcriptome sequencing, which achieves diagnostic yields of 10% to 35%. International-scale collaboration and establishment of data repositories are paramount in accelerating the diagnosis of Mendelian disorders.

> A combination of different types of evidence incorporating population data, functional studies, clinical data, and predictive tools is necessary for thorough, thoughtful variant classification. Variant classification criteria may be optimized in a quantitative, gene-specific manner using validated predictors of pathogenicity for genes or conditions with sufficient information. Large-scale data (genome sequencing of healthy and affected cohorts, high-throughput functional studies, and in silico metapredictors) increase the robustness of evidence used for variant classification and

lend themselves to incorporation in quantitative frameworks. Collaborative efforts by laboratories and disease-specific expert groups reduce variant classification discrepancies and improve the quality of variant interpretation information available to patients and researchers.

Clinical bioinformatics system is well-established for diagnosing genetic disease based on next-generation sequencing, but requires special considerations when being adapted for the next-generation sequencing-based genetic diagnosis of mitochondrial diseases. Challenges are caused by the involvement of mitochondrial DNA genome in disease etiology. Heteroplasmy and haplogroup are key factors in interpreting mitochondrial DNA variant effects. Data resources and tools for analyzing variant and sequencing data are available at MSeqDR, MitoMap, and HmtDB. Revised specifications of the American College of Medical Genetics/Association of Molecular Pathology standards and guidelines for mitochondrial DNA variant interpretation are proposed by the MSeqDr Consortium and community experts.

Clinical bioinformatics encompasses generating raw sequence data from the machine through identifying reportable variants. Throughout the process, important quality control metrics are tracked based on the data, including the completeness of coverage across the region of interest for the assay. The process starts by taking raw sequence data, aligning it to a reference genome, and identifying variants based on the quality of the reads and the base pair calls. Variants are then annotated and filtered using a variety of features, including gene, transcript, Human Genome Variation Society nomenclature, population frequency, and presence in databases. In a clinical setting, a thorough validation of each of the components of the bioinformatics pipeline is critical, as is a detailed understanding of infrastructure, privacy, and security requirements.

Inherited retinal diseases (IRDs) represent a diverse array of conditions characterized by dysfunction or loss of 1 or more retinal cell types. Next-generation sequencing has enabled rapid and relatively inexpensive genotyping, with more than 250 genes identified as responsible for IRDs. This expansion in molecular diagnostic accuracy, in combination with the retina's relative accessibility and immune privilege, has fostered the development of precision therapies to treat these myriad conditions. Novel techniques are being used in early trials. Precision molecular therapies for IRDs hold great promise as diagnostic and treatment strategies continue to expand.

Therapeutic gene editing with the clustered regularly interspaced short palindromic repeat (CRISPR)–Cas system offers significant improvements in specificity and programmability compared with previous methods. CRISPR editing strategies can be used ex vivo and in vivo with many theoretic disease applications. Off-target effects of CRISPR-mediated gene editing are an important outcome to be aware of, minimize, and detect. The current methods of regulatory approval for personalized therapies are complex and may be proved inefficient as these therapies are implemented more widely. The role of pathologists and laboratory medicine practitioners is vital to the clinical implementation of therapeutic gene editing.

Whole-genome sequencing (WGS) identifies critical alterations in the genome that are not present in the coding genes. Genome-wide methylation studies identify epi-signatures that allow clarification and proper classification of variants of uncertain significance. RNA-seq, both targeted and untargeted, allows diagnosis of human disorders, particularly those in patients with a suspicious phenotype and no obvious genomic alteration. Bioinformatics tools, and neural networks, allow for the association of apparently unrelated events. Multi-omic analysis—the integrated analysis of data from various omic studies (WGS, methylation, RNAseq)—identifies coordinated interaction of variants leading to a phenotype.

CLINICS IN LABORATORY MEDICINE

SERIES OF RELATED INTEREST

Surgical Pathology Clinics
Available at: https://www.surgpath.theclinics.com/

THE CLINICS ARE NOW AVAILABLE ONLINE!
Access your subscription at:
www.theclinics.com

Preface

Precision Medicine Exits the Hype Cycle and Enters into Productive Clinical Use

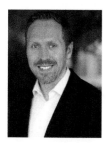

Ryan J. Schmidt, MD, PhD
Editor

The notion of precision medicine broadly refers to the administration of a patient-specific treatment based on unique features of an individual or their disease that are identified in the laboratory. This concept is not new to medicine and has existed for many years to allow for the administration of compatible blood products and antibiotics selected based on antibiotic resistance testing. The modern incarnation of precision medicine leverages our ability to determine the molecular cause of genetic disorders and apply rational therapies based on specific disease-causing genetic variants.

Technological advances in molecular genetics have rapidly increased our understanding of constitutional genetic disorders. Broad-based clinical molecular diagnostic testing has now become standard in many disease areas. The results of this testing now have the potential to extend beyond providing a diagnosis and serve as a basis for precision therapies that target specific genetic alterations. In addition, clinical molecular diagnostic testing can serve as a starting point for additional research that increases our understanding of genetic disease. Collectively, these components comprise the foundation for a comprehensive precision medicine program. The combination of diagnosis, treatment, and research capabilities has the potential to interact in a synergistic manner when thoughtfully implemented together at a single institution.

As the precision medicine enterprise matures, it faces a variety of barriers that currently limit its widespread use. Now that the technical challenges that surround developing and implementing a precision therapy are being overcome, the financial and regulatory components of this model of care must also be built.

Precision medicine has begun to exit the hype cycle and enter into productive clinical use. As we celebrate the treatment of the first patients with precision therapies, we must consider what it will take to diagnose and treat the last patients with the most

Clin Lab Med 40 (2020) ix–x
https://doi.org/10.1016/j.cll.2020.04.001
0272-2712/20/© 2020 Published by Elsevier Inc.

technically challenging genetic variants. In addition, we must address the needs to effectively scale up the precision medicine enterprise and overcome the practical barriers that will inhibit the widespread application of these complementary diagnostic and therapeutic approaches.

Ryan J. Schmidt, MD, PhD
Clinical Genomics Laboratory
Center for Personalized Medicine
Department of Pathology and
Laboratory Medicine
Children's Hospital Los Angeles
Keck School of Medicine of USC
2100 West 3rd Street, Suite 300
Los Angeles, CA 90057, USA

E-mail address:
rschmidt@chla.usc.edu

Enhancing Diagnosis Through RNA Sequencing

David R. Murdock, MD

KEYWORDS

- RNA sequencing (RNAseq) • Exome sequencing (ES) • Genome sequencing (GS)
- Variants of uncertain significance (VUS) • Noncoding variation

KEY POINTS

- The diagnostic rate of exome and genome sequencing remains only 25% to 30%, due in part to the difficulty in interpreting variants of uncertain significance and noncoding mutations.
- RNA sequencing (RNAseq) reveals the functional consequence of genetic variation through the detection of abnormal gene expression levels, differences in gene splicing, and allele specific expression.
- RNAseq increases the diagnostic rate by 7.5% to 36% depending on disease type and tissue source.
- Gene expression is tissue specific. Blood and skin fibroblasts are most common tissue sources but may not be suitable for all diseases.

INTRODUCTION

The widespread utilization of exome sequencing (ES) and genome sequencing (GS) has transformed diagnostic capabilities for suspected rare Mendelian disorders. In addition, large gene panels are now frequently sent for patients with suspected genetic conditions, including hereditary cancer syndromes, hyperlipidemias, and aortopathies. Many patients undergoing ES and GS still remain undiagnosed with most studies reporting diagnostic rates of only 25% to 30%.[1,2] Although the application of ES, GS, and gene panels has transformed diagnostic capabilities for genetic diseases, a substantial challenge exists in the interpretation of variants of uncertain significance (VUS), the role of noncoding mutations, and the downstream mechanistic consequences of these and other genetic changes. RNA sequencing (RNAseq) is now emerging as an adjunct to DNA sequencing with the potential to further improve diagnostic capabilities and guide management by revealing the functional consequence of detected genetic variants. RNAseq is an extremely powerful method for

Department of Molecular and Human Genetics, Baylor College of Medicine, One Baylor Plaza, BCM225, Houston, TX 77030, USA
E-mail address: drmurdoc@bcm.edu

Clin Lab Med 40 (2020) 113–119
https://doi.org/10.1016/j.cll.2020.02.001
0272-2712/20/© 2020 Elsevier Inc. All rights reserved.

labmed.theclinics.com

analyzing the transcriptome to detect alterations at the RNA level that may have therapeutic, diagnostic, and prognostic significance.

RNA SEQUENCING METHODOLOGY

RNAseq is based on the same underlying next-generation sequencing (NGS) methods used in ES/GS (**Fig. 1**). The first step in this process involves the collection and isolation of RNA (transcriptome) from a particular tissue source. The choice of tissue is important because not every gene is expressed in all tissues, and not every tissue is easily accessible. The most commonly used tissues for RNAseq are blood and fibroblasts, the latter usually derived from skin biopsy samples. The next step involves the conversion of RNA (typically messenger RNA [mRNA]) fragments into complementary DNA (cDNA) via reverse transcription, generating what is known as a cDNA library. This collection of cDNA is then sequenced via NGS technology, typically using Illumina short read sequencing, producing millions of reads that are then aligned to a reference genome for additional downstream analysis. Unlike DNA sequencing that is focused on only the nucleotide sequences, RNAseq also provides the ability to detect abnormal gene expression levels, differences in gene splicing, allele specific expression (ASE), and other transcriptomic information.

GENE EXPRESSION

A common genetic disease mechanism involves gene expression outside of the normal physiologic range. In many cases, abnormally low levels of expression lead to disease where a single functional copy of a gene does not produce enough gene product (ie, haploinsufficiency). For example, Lynch syndrome and its associated risk of colorectal and other cancers is frequently due to loss-of-function (LOF) variants in mismatch repair genes that result in decreased expression of genes that are necessary for DNA repair.[3] Although DNA sequencing can be used to identify LOF variants,

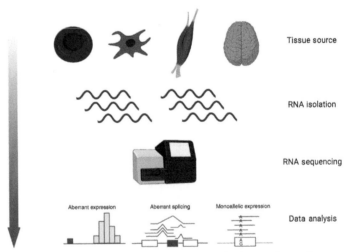

Fig. 1. Steps involved in RNAseq. First, the tissue source is chosen depending on availability and disease class. Then RNA is isolated and converted to cDNA via a reverse transcriptase followed by sequencing on NGS platform. Finally, sequencing reads are aligned, and downstream analysis is performed to identify abnormal gene expression, gene splicing, and ASE. (*Adapted from* Kremer LS, Bader DM, Mertes C, et al. Genetic diagnosis of Mendelian disorders via RNA sequencing. Nat Commun. 2017;8:3; with permission.)

such as nonsense and frameshift insertion/deletions that lead to haploinsufficiency, it is much more difficult to predict the effect of variants in promoters, enhancers, introns, or even coding missense variants that may influence gene expression. In RNAseq, however, expression levels are directly measured by counting the number of reads mapping to each gene. By comparing this number to a control data set, it is possible to detect expression outliers that may be clinically relevant. Such techniques have been used to identify the genetic cause in patients with mitochondrial disorders where ES was unrevealing.[4]

GENE SPLICING

Normal gene splicing is a critical step in the production of proteins. This process involves the removal of noncoding introns and joining of exons from pre-mRNA before protein synthesis.[5] Defects in gene splicing can result in disease via several mechanisms that include exon skipping, exon extension, intron retention, or creation of new exons[5,6] (**Fig. 2**).

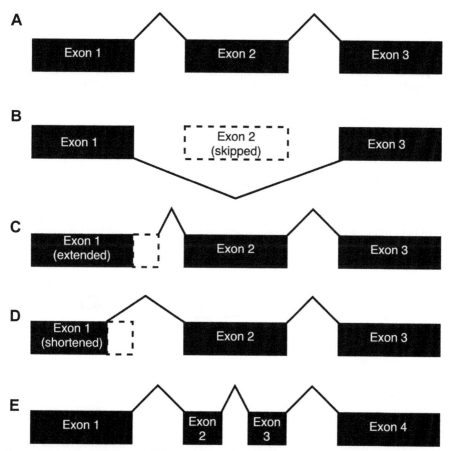

Fig. 2. Types of alternative splicing events. (*A*) Normal exon splicing. (*B*) Exon 2 skipped because of canonical splice site variant. (*C*) Exon 1 extension because of cryptic splice site activation within intron. (*D*) Exon 1 shortening because of cryptic splice site activation within exon. (*E*) Mutually exclusive exons.

Abnormal splicing of the same gene can even give rise to different phenotypes. Duchenne muscular dystrophy is frequently caused by splicing variants that cause exon skipping and resulting frameshifts leading to complete lack of dystrophin expression.[5–7] In contrast, Becker muscular dystrophy may result from splice site variants that cause in-frame exon skipping and abnormal but present dystrophin.[5–7]

Intronic variants within 1 or 2 nucleotides from an exon, the canonical splice sites, are typically considered pathogenic.[8] In contrast, the effect of intronic variants outside this region that could activate a cryptic splice site is difficult to predict.[5] A recent review by Vaz-Drago and colleagues[9] identified 185 disease-associated deep intronic variants in 77 different genes leading to such disorders as cystic fibrosis, Fabry disease, and familial adenomatous polyposis. Similarly, the consequence of synonymous variants whereby the encoded amino acid is the same but RNA splicing may be abnormal is uncertain without transcriptomic information.[6] Hutchinson-Gilford progeria syndrome is due to a de novo synonymous variant in *LMNA* (c.1824C>T) that does not change the translated glycine amino acid (p.Gly608=) but activates a cryptic splice site resulting in a truncated and dysfunctional protein and features of accelerated aging.[10] Other examples include the "silent" change in *FBN1*, c.6354C>T (p.Ile2118=), causing Marfan syndrome, and in the mismatch repair gene *MSH2*, c.2634G>A (p.Glu878=), leading to Lynch syndrome and a greatly increased risk of colorectal, endometrial, and other cancers.[11,12] Fresard and colleagues recently identified a synonymous variant, c.456G>T (p.Val152=), in the epilepsy gene *KCTD7* in a 12-year-old girl with developmental regression and seizures.[13] RNAseq from blood demonstrated that this change created a new splicing junction resulting in exon truncation (**Fig. 3**). The variant and splicing defect segregated with other affected family members and was presumed to be the cause of the proband's neurologic phenotype.

Several in silico tools, such as ESEfinder,[14] MaxEnt,[15] and Human Splicing Finder,[16] exist to estimate splicing impact in the absence of transcriptomic information. However, these models have significant false positive rates and other limitations that limit their usefulness.[17] Recently, a novel artificial intelligence (AI) tool, SpliceAI, was developed to predict whether noncoding genetic variants cause cryptic splicing using a deep learning network.[18] According to Jaganathan and colleagues,[18] 75% of predicted cryptic splice variants validated on RNAseq, which represents a great improvement over other algorithms. These predictions, however, still need to be functionally

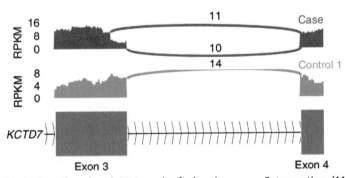

Fig. 3. Sashimi plot of proband RNAseq (*red*) showing exon 3 truncation (11/21 reads) because of germline synonymous variant in *KCTD7*. Normal splicing in control sample (*blue*). RPKM, reads per kilobase million. (*Adapted from* Frésard L, Smail C, Ferraro NM, et al. Identification of rare-disease genes using blood transcriptome sequencing and large control cohorts. Nat Med. 2019;25(6):911-9; with permission.)

validated before they can be used as support for pathogenicity. In contrast, RNAseq is able to identify aberrant splicing by detecting abnormal splicing isoforms directly.

ALLELE-SPECIFIC EXPRESSION

RNAseq can also show evidence of ASE in which only 1 allele is expressed while the other is silenced.[4] Such monoallelic expression can occur for several reasons, including imprinting, nonsense mediated decay, or regulatory effects leading to selective allele expression.[19] Evidence of ASE is especially helpful in prioritizing variants when only a single pathogenic heterozygous variant is identified on DNA sequencing but a recessive mode of inheritance is suspected.[4] Kremer and colleagues[4] diagnosed 2 patients with a mitochondrial proline metabolism defect and a mucolipidosis, both autosomal recessive conditions, by identifying ASE in the *ALDH18A1* and *MCOLN1* gene, respectively.

VARIANT OF UNCERTAIN SIGNIFICANCE RESOLUTION

In 2015, the American College of Medical Genetics and Genomics (ACMG) and Association for Molecular Pathology published guidelines for interpretation of sequencing variants.[8] These guidelines have been an immense step forward in the standardization of variant interpretation because they provide rules used to classify variants (eg, benign or pathogenic). However, if insufficient evidence is available to make a final determination, variants fall into the uncertain significance category, and their clinical impact remains unknown. Variants of uncertain significance (VUS) pose a challenge for medical practice because they are neither a positive nor a negative result that would clearly dictate management strategies. It is not recommended that a VUS be used for clinical decision making, but instead management should be based on personal and family history only.[8] Unfortunately, up to one-third of patients undergoing germline cancer genetic testing have at least 1 VUS identified.[20,21] Furthermore, the number of VUS increases with number of genes sequenced,[22,23] demonstrating a major drawback to sending large gene panels or even clinical ES/GS. In addition, the ACMG guidelines focus on coding changes, leaving most noncoding variants detected on ES/GS in the VUS category. In addition, because variant classification relies heavily on population-specific allele frequencies, patients of non-European ancestry are more likely to receive VUS results than others.[23]

RNAseq can be used to reclassify VUS, for example, when a splicing effect is predicted but outside the canonical splice site. In 1 study from a major clinical laboratory performing hereditary cancer testing, supplementing DNA sequencing with RNAseq resulted in resolution of 88% of VUS that potentially affected splicing.[17] In particular, 47% of these VUS were upgraded to likely pathogenic, whereas 41% were downgraded to benign, resulting in significant clinical management changes for these patients and their families.[17] Other studies have shown that RNAseq increases the diagnostic rate of unsolved cases between 7.5% and 36% above the baseline 25% to 30% normally provided by ES and GS alone.[1,2,4,13,19,24] In particular, the ability to rule in or out noncoding variants detected on GS is particularly powerful given that these would likely remain VUS without additional functional context.

LIMITATIONS

Despite its many applications, there are still limitations to the widespread application of RNAseq. One major challenge is that gene expression varies significantly between different tissues. The Genotype-Tissue Expression Consortium (GTEx) was established to create a reference dataset of tissue-specific gene expression and regulation.[25] RNAseq samples from 54 different tissue types across nearly 1000 individuals were collected by GTEx. One can search GTEx to determine which genes are expressed at sufficient levels in specific tissues to obtain adequate results from RNAseq. However, this requires prior identification of candidate genes, something not possible for novel disease genes.

Another major limitation of RNAseq as it is currently practiced is that the optimal RNA source is frequently not easily accessible.[4,19,24,26] Although RNA derived from blood and skin fibroblasts is relatively simple to collect, other tissues, such as brain or muscle, require much more invasive collection techniques. Blood is generally considered the least informative of tissues with a recent study using blood transcriptome data demonstrating only a 7.5% diagnostic rate.[13] In fact, the genes most commonly associated with muscle disease have low expression in blood, making it an inadequate tissue source for neuromuscular conditions.[26] The differentiation of accessible cells (eg, skin fibroblasts) into specific cell types (eg, neurons) will likely be needed to overcome this tissue-specific expression limitation.[27]

SUMMARY

In this era of precision medicine and expanded genetic testing, the need to understand the functional consequences of genetic variation will become even more important. For example, the National Institutes of Health–funded All of Us research study will perform GS on 1,000,000+ people in the United States over the next 5 years, generating an enormous amount of genomic data, much of which will be in difficult-to-interpret regions of the genome. Clinical GS will replace ES in the coming years as costs fall and the quest for improving diagnostic rates continues. RNAseq is an effective tool for assessing the transcriptional consequences of a wide variety of DNA variants, both coding and noncoding. Although challenges remain, RNAseq offers a powerful tool to improve diagnostic rates and understand disease mechanisms.

DISCLOSURE

The author has nothing to disclose.

REFERENCES

1. Yang Y, Muzny DM, Xia F, et al. Molecular findings among patients referred for clinical whole-exome sequencing. JAMA 2014;312(18):1870–9.
2. Posey JE, Rosenfeld JA, James RA, et al. Molecular diagnostic experience of whole-exome sequencing in adult patients. Genet Med 2016;18(7):678–85.
3. Kohlmann W, Gruber SB. Lynch syndrome. 1993. Available at: http://www.ncbi.nlm.nih.gov/pubmed/20301390.
4. Kremer LS, Bader DM, Mertes C, et al. Genetic diagnosis of Mendelian disorders via RNA sequencing. Nat Commun 2017;8:1–11.
5. Scotti MM, Swanson MS. RNA mis-splicing in disease. Nat Rev Genet 2016;17(1):19–32.
6. Anna A, Monika G. Splicing mutations in human genetic disorders: examples, detection, and confirmation. J Appl Genet 2018;59(3):253–68.
7. Darras BT, Urion DK, Ghosh PS. Dystrophinopathies. 1993. Available at: http://www.ncbi.nlm.nih.gov/pubmed/20301298.
8. Richards S, Aziz N, Bale S, et al. Standards and guidelines for the interpretation of sequence variants: a joint consensus recommendation of the American

College of Medical Genetics and Genomics and the Association for Molecular Pathology. Genet Med 2015;17(5):405–24.

9. Vaz-Drago R, Custódio N, Carmo-Fonseca M. Deep intronic mutations and human disease. Hum Genet 2017;136(9):1093–111.

10. Eriksson M, Brown WT, Gordon LB, et al. Recurrent de novo point mutations in lamin A cause Hutchinson-Gilford progeria syndrome. Nature 2003;423(6937): 293–8.

11. Liu W, Qian C, Francke U. Silent mutation induces exon skipping of fibrillin-1 gene in Marfan syndrome. Nat Genet 1997;16(4):328–9.

12. Pérez-Cabornero L, Infante M, Velasco E, et al. Evaluating the effect of unclassified variants identified in MMR genes using phenotypic features, bioinformatics prediction, and RNA assays. J Mol Diagn 2013;15(3):380–90.

13. Frésard L, Smai C, Ferraro NM, et al. Identification of rare-disease genes using blood transcriptome sequencing and large control cohorts. Nat Med 2019; 25(6):911–9.

14. Cartegni L, Wang J, Zhu Z, et al. ESEfinder: a web resource to identify exonic splicing enhancers. Nucleic Acids Res 2003;31(13):3568–71.

15. Yeo G, Burge CB. Maximum entropy modeling of short sequence motifs with applications to RNA splicing signals. J Comput Biol 2004;11(2–3):377–94.

16. Desmet F-O, Hamroun D, Lalande M, et al. Human splicing finder: an online bioinformatics tool to predict splicing signals. Nucleic Acids Res 2009;37(9):e67.

17. Karam R, Conner B, LaDuca H, et al. Assessment of diagnostic outcomes of RNA genetic testing for hereditary cancer. JAMA Netw Open 2019;2(10):e1913900.

18. Jaganathan K, Kyriazopoulou Panagiotopoulou S, McRae JF, et al. Predicting splicing from primary sequence with deep learning. Cell 2019;176(3): 535–48.e24.

19. Lee H, Huang AY, Wang L-K, et al. Diagnostic utility of transcriptome sequencing for rare Mendelian diseases. Genet Med 2019. https://doi.org/10.1038/s41436-019-0672-1.

20. LaDuca H, Stuenkel AJ, Dolinsky JS, et al. Utilization of multigene panels in hereditary cancer predisposition testing: analysis of more than 2,000 patients. Genet Med 2014;16(11):830–7.

21. Tung N, Lin NU, Kidd J, et al. Frequency of germline mutations in 25 cancer susceptibility genes in a sequential series of patients with breast cancer. J Clin Oncol 2016;34(13):1460–8.

22. Wong EK, Bartels K, Hathaway J, et al. Perceptions of genetic variant reclassification in patients with inherited cardiac disease. Eur J Hum Genet 2019;27(7): 1134–42.

23. Caswell-Jin JL, Gupta T, Hall E, et al. Racial/ethnic differences in multiple-gene sequencing results for hereditary cancer risk. Genet Med 2018;20(2):234–9.

24. Cummings BB, Marshall JL, Tukiainen T, et al. Improving genetic diagnosis in Mendelian disease with transcriptome sequencing. Sci Transl Med 2017; 9(386):1–25.

25. GTEx Consortium. The Genotype-Tissue Expression (GTEx) project. Nat Genet 2013;45(6):580–5.

26. Gonorazky HD, Naumenko S, Ramani AK, et al. Expanding the boundaries of RNA sequencing as a diagnostic tool for rare Mendelian disease. Am J Hum Genet 2019;104(3):466–83.

27. Tsunemoto RK, Eade KT, Blanchard JW, et al. Forward engineering neuronal diversity using direct reprogramming. EMBO J 2015;34(11):1445–55.

The Clinical Application of RNA Sequencing in Genetic Diagnosis of Mendelian Disorders

Sarah L. Stenton, MBChB, MPhil[a,b],*, Holger Prokisch, PhD[a,b]

KEYWORDS

- RNA-seq • Genomic sequencing • Variant prioritization • Diagnostic yield

KEY POINTS

- Molecular genetic approaches have evolved at an astonishing pace resulting in increasingly routine use of whole exome sequencing in Mendelian disorder diagnosis.
- After whole exome sequencing, 50% to 75% of patients remain without a genetic diagnosis, indicating limitations in variant calling and prioritization and a role for noncoding variants.
- Whole genome sequencing has the potential to reveal all genetic variants; however, it escalates the challenge of variant prioritization owing to the vast numbers called.
- Promising approaches to aid in variant interpretation include the integration of functional genomic data such as transcriptome sequencing, which achieves diagnostic yields of 10% to 35%.
- International-scale collaboration and establishment of data repositories are paramount in accelerating the diagnosis of Mendelian disorders.

INTRODUCTION

Molecular genetic approaches have evolved at astonishing pace in capacity, capability, and application in recent years, reflected by the increasingly routine use of whole

This article originally appeared in *Advances in Molecular Pathology*, Volume 1, 2018.
Disclosure Statement: The authors have nothing to declare.
Funding: mitoNet German Network for Mitochondrial Diseases (01GM1113). GENOMIT European Network for Mitochondrial Disease (01GM1207). SOUND (Statistical Multi-Omics Understanding) EU Horizon2020 Collaborative Research Project (633974). PhD Program Medical Life Science and Technology scholarship (TUM School of Medicine).
[a] Institute of Human Genetics, Klinikum rechts der Isar, Technische Universität München, Ismaninger Straße 22, 81675, Munich, Germany; [b] Institute of Human Genetics, Helmholtz Zentrum München, Ingolstaedter Landstraße 1, 85764, Neuherberg, Germany
* Corresponding author. Institute of Human Genetics (IHG), Helmholtz Zentrum München, Deutsches Forschungszentrum für Gesundheit und Umwelt (GmbH), Building 3537, Room 8128, Ingolstaedter Landstr. 1, Neuherberg D-85764, Germany.
E-mail address: sarah.stenton@helmholtz-muenchen.de

exome sequencing (WES) in Mendelian and rare disorder diagnosis[1–3] and by the approximately 160 new disease–gene discoveries documented yearly.[4] However, despite the revolutionary ascension of WES, 50% to 75% of patients remain without a genetic diagnosis (**Fig. 1**)[5–8] and, furthermore, more than 3000 Mendelian disorders are yet to be genetically defined.[8] This diagnostic rate may seems to be low. However, these figures must be considered in the context of the inability of WES to appreciate the impact of variation outside of the exonic regions. WES covers just 2% of the genome,[9] the exonic protein-coding regions, indicating that disease-causing variants may be harboring in the noncoding regions, such as deep intronic or regulatory variants.[10]

By contrast, whole genome sequencing (WGS) has the potential to capture nearly all genomic variation in an unbiased manner, with higher sensitivity than WES for certain coding variants, indels, copy number variants, and chromosomal rearrangements.[11–13] Additionally, WGS reveals variants in the regulatory noncoding regions and more complex rearrangements, such as inversions and transposons.[14] In terms of influence on diagnostic rate, WGS has been reported to identify disease-causing variants in an additional 14% compared with WES, with an overall diagnostic yield of 41%.[15]

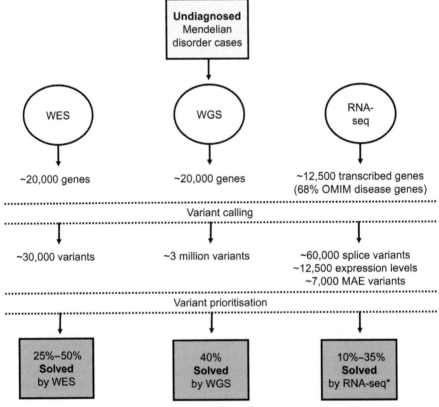

Fig. 1. Schematic of the analysis pipeline for whole exome sequencing (WES), whole genome sequencing (WGS), and transcriptome sequencing (RNA-seq) with the number of genes and variants and the currently reported diagnostic yield. *Unsolved WES cases. MAE, monoallelic expression.

However, WGS increases the challenge of variant prioritization owing to the sizable number of variants called (approximately 3 million).[7,16,17] The former challenge of variant discovery has, therefore, shifted to the ability to interpret function and ultimately clinical impact of such variants,[18–20] rendering numerous disease-causing variants to be variants of unknown significance (VUS).

A promising approach to aid in variant interpretation is the integration of functional genomic data such as the transcriptome.[21,22] Transcriptome sequencing (RNA-seq) has already proven useful in elucidating mechanisms of cancer and common disease,[23–25] but until recently had not been systematically applied in Mendelian disorder diagnosis.

THE CHALLENGE OF VARIANT CALLING AND PRIORITIZATION

Variant calling and prioritization play central roles in genomic sequencing analysis. Sequencing error resulting in artifactual data is a common phenomenon and, owing to the diversity in variant calling algorithms and filtering strategies as well as the aspiration for high sensitivity and precision, distinguishing low-frequency potentially disease-causing variants from random sequencing errors remains a significant challenge.[26] Variant prioritization, defined as the process of determining whether identified variants have the potential to damage gene function and thus underlie disease phenotype,[27] aims to ultimately identify the 1 to 2 variants responsible for a patient's Mendelian disorder. This is a classic needle in the haystack problem,[28] approached by enforcing filters for inheritance model, minimum population allele frequency (according to population-scale variation databases, such as the Exome Aggregation Consortium,[29] the Genome Aggregation Database, and the 1000 Genomes Project)[16] and variant effect. Numerous variant effect prediction tools can be used; however, those for noncoding variants remain less accurate than their protein-coding counterparts, owing to insufficient understanding of the regulatory machinery encrypted in noncoding DNA.[27] Thus, reinforcing the argument for integration of functional transcriptomic (RNA-seq) data.

THE TRANSCRIPTOME AND RNA-SEQ

The transcriptome describes the complete set of transcripts in a cell and their abundance for a specific snapshot in time.[30] In contrast with DNA, which is essentially identical across all cells, the actively transcribed RNA is highly dynamic, serving as a transient intermediary molecule between DNA and protein translation, therefore, revealing the link between the cellular phenotype and the underpinning genetics.[25]

RNA-seq is the first genome scale sequencing methodology to allow the entire transcriptome to be surveyed in a high-throughput, quantitative, and qualitative manner. It has emerged as a part of the development of NGS technologies, with the capability to both quantify known predefined RNA species and to detect and quantify rare and novel RNA transcript variants and isoforms,[31] thus, providing a direct insight into the transcriptional perturbations caused by VUS (frequently synonymous or noncoding variants) such as on RNA abundance and isoform.[32]

RNA-SEQ METHODOLOGY

RNA-seq is not a single protocol, but rather a workflow of methodologies encompassing sample preparation, sequencing, and downstream computational analysis.[25] First, cells are disrupted for isolation of RNA. Owing to the inherent labile nature of RNA, degradation and subsequent low input amounts[33] are considerable challenges, addressed by optimizing protocols for the input of just 0.1 to 1.0 μg of total high-quality RNA (RNA integrity number of >8).[34] Second, library preparation is required. An umbrella term for the purification and enrichment of messenger RNA by selection of Poly(A)+ transcripts and/or depletion of contaminating ribosomal RNA, fragmentation (necessitated by the size limitation of sequencing platforms), amplification by polymerase chain reaction (to ensure sufficient coverage of the transcriptome and to enable detection of low abundance transcripts) and finally cDNA synthesis and sequencing.[25] A nonstranded or stranded protocol can be used in the cDNA synthesis step of library preparation (**Fig. 2**). The more recently developed stranded methods allow retention of information on which strand the messenger RNA template originated, thus, allowing determination of expression from genes with overlapping genomic coordinates but transcription from opposite strands.[35] The leading protocol, dUTP second-strand marking, uses dUTPs instead of dTTPs during the synthesis of the second strand cDNA.[36] Marking of the second strand cDNA with uracils permits degradation with uracil-DNA-glycosylase, facilitating the preservation of strand-of-origin information during adapter ligation and library enrichment by polymerase chain reaction. After quality control measures, the short-read data require computational reconstruction of the original RNA transcript by alignment of reads to the human reference genome to detect and measure expression.[37]

INTERPRETATION OF RNA-SEQ

The analysis of RNA-seq data in the context of Mendelian disorders is a novel and developing field. At present, 3 situations can be interpreted to prioritize candidate disease-causing variants for rare Mendelian disorders[21] (**Fig. 3**). First, RNA-seq can reveal extreme cases of allele-specific expression, termed monoallelic expression (MAE), whereby 1 allele is silenced, leaving only the other allele expressed (see **Fig. 3**A). When assuming an autosomal recessive mode of inheritance, genes with a

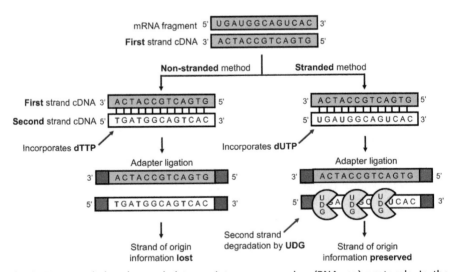

Fig. 2. Nonstranded and stranded transcriptome sequencing (RNA-seq) protocols. In the stranded protocol, during cDNA synthesis, second strand synthesis utilizes dUTPs in place of dTTPs with subsequent second strand degradation by uracil-DNA-glycosylase. This ensures that strand of origin information during adapter ligation and library enrichment by polymerase chain reaction is preserved.

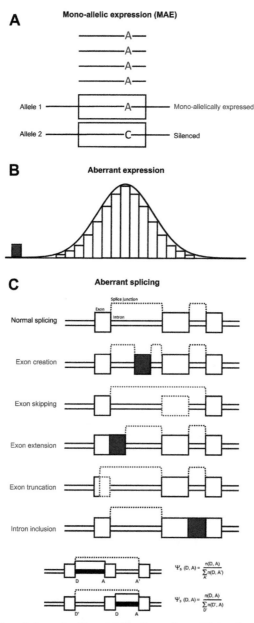

Fig. 3. Three situations interpreted in prioritization of candidate disease-causing variants for rare Mendelian disorders. (*A*) Monoallelic expression (MAE), (*B*) aberrant expression, and (*C*) aberrant splicing. Frequency of splice variants is calculated by the percent spliced in (psi) denoted by ψ. The ψ_5-splicing index defines the number of reads supporting the splicing event from D to A relative to the combined number of reads supporting splicing from D to any acceptor site A'. The ψ_3-splicing index defines the number of reads supporting the splicing event from D to A relative to the combined number of reads supporting splicing from any donor site D' to A.[52] Aberrant expression or splicing is defined as statistically significant deviation from the normal distribution of the controls.

single heterozygous rare coding variant (minor allele frequency of <0.01) identified by WES analysis are not prioritized. However, MAE of such variants fits the recessive mode of inheritance assumption. Detection of MAE can thus help in reprioritizing heterozygous rare variants.

MAE can arise as a consequence of multiple mechanisms, encompassing allele-specific transcription, genomic imprinting and X-chromosome inactivation.[38,39] Genomic imprinting is the most frequent mechanism, whereby DNA methylation and histone modifications result in biased expression of an allele in a parent-of-origin–specific manner, exemplified in Angelman syndrome owing to deficient maternal allele expression of *UBE3A* in the brain.[40] Additionally, posttranscriptional mechanisms can result in MEA, such as alternative splicing causing exon skipping and MEA of variants contained within the skipped exon[41] and such as the creation of premature stop codons leading to nonsense-mediated decay of one allele and MAE of the other.[21,42,43]

Second, genes with expression outside physiologic range can be identified as expression outliers (see **Fig. 3**B), termed aberrant expression. The cause of such aberrant expression includes rare variants in promoter and enhancer regions[44] and rare variants within both coding and intronic regions[24], in addition to posttranscriptional mechanisms.

Third, splicing of a gene can be affected (see **Fig. 3**C). Aberrant splicing has long been recognized as a major cause of Mendelian disorders[45–47] and, in fact, approximately 10% of exonic disease-associated alleles are found to disrupt splicing.[48] Any change in exonic sequence may disrupt or create cis-acting elements, which facilitate exon recognition, resulting in aberrant splicing. Splice-disrupting variants may also be located in the deep intronic sequence[49] and thus not covered by WES or detected by WGS, but not prioritized. Hence, direct probing of splice isoforms by RNA-seq is important and can detect an array of splice defects from exon creation, skipping, extension, and truncation to intronic inclusion, providing invaluable information about exonic and intronic positions susceptible to affect splicing. Aberrant splicing events can be detected by testing for differential splicing between an individual case and a control population. Splice sites can be annotated with reference exon annotation such as provided by GENCODE.[50] Detection of de novo splice sites, however, requires the use of annotation-free algorithms, such as provided by the LeafCutter software.[51]

SYSTEMATIC ANALYSIS OF RNA-SEQ IN MENDELIAN DISORDER DIAGNOSIS

In parallel effort, 2 studies systematically investigated the use of RNA-seq for the molecular genetic diagnosis of Mendelian disorders, using near analogous approaches[21,22] (**Table 1**).

Table 1
The Diagnostic Yield of WES and RNA-Seq Analyses in Mendelian Disorders

Patient Cohort	Total Cases	Undiagnosed Cases	Diagnostic Yield of WES	Diagnostic Yield of RNA-Seq
Mitochondrial disorders (Kremer et al,[21] 2017)	105	48	35% to 60%[10,53–56]	5/48 (10%)
Rare muscle disorders (Cummings et al,[22] 2017)	63	50	25% to 50%[5–8]	17/50 (35%)

Abbreviation: WES, whole exome sequencing.

RNA-SEQ IN UNDIAGNOSED MITOCHONDRIAL DISORDERS

Kremer and colleagues[21] investigated the application of RNA-seq in 105 mitochondrial disorder cases, a clinically and genetically heterogeneous cohort of patients with a rare disorder, of whom only 35% to 60%[10,53–56] receive a diagnosis after WES. Mitochondrial disorders have a complex genetic architecture with more than 1500 genes implicated in healthy mitochondrial function[57] and causal defects identified in more than 300 genes implicated in mitochondrial metabolism.[58] An additional layer of complexity arises from the bigenomic control of the energy-generating oxidative phosphorylation system, primarily responsible for mitochondrial disorders, and disrupted by both mitochondrial DNA and nuclear DNA variants.[59] Despite disease manifestation occurring in the high-energy demanding tissues (such as brain, heart, muscle, and liver) for which biopsy is often unobtainable, skin biopsy and thus fibroblast cell lines allow mitochondrial disease mechanisms to be assayed.[60] Fibroblasts are, therefore, a readily available resource for RNA-seq analysis and for downstream rapid demonstration of the role of candidate variants by complementation assays.[61]

There were 105 fibroblast cell lines that were analyzed, 48 for which WES did not yield a diagnosis. Genetically diagnosed patients were included in the analysis pipeline to increase the power for the detection of aberrant events. The study considered all transcribed genes in the fibroblast cell lines and, after filtering to remove lowly expressed genes, identified 12,680 transcribed genes. The genetic variants were systemically prioritized with 3 strategies: MAE, defined as 80% or greater of transcripts harboring the rare variant of a heterozygous single nucleotide polymorphism, aberrant expression, and aberrant splicing. Read count outliers (aberrant expression) were identified as those with an absolute Z-score of greater than 3 and statistical significance according to DESeq2, a statistical test originally developed for differential expression analysis[62] that is applied by testing each sample in turn against the remainder. The analysis of aberrant splicing used an annotation-free algorithm comparing the percentage of splice variants at each exon between one patient and the remainder to detect spice outliers from the normal distribution. This method allowed each to serve as a control for one another, a robust strategy given the genetic diversity in mitochondrial disorders.[21]

The method resulted in the median detection of 6 monoallelically expressed rare variants, 1 aberrantly expressed gene, and 5 aberrant splicing events per case. Notably, among the 175 aberrantly spliced genes detected, the most abundant events were the differential expression of isoforms, exon skipping, and the creation of new exons. This resulted in an overall molecular genetic diagnosis of 10% of patients with undiagnosed mitochondriopathy (5 of 48) and a yield of promising candidate genes for 36 additional patients.[21]

RNA-SEQ IN UNDIAGNOSED PRIMARY MUSCLE DISORDERS

Cummings and colleagues[22] investigated the application of RNA-seq in 63 rare muscle disorder cases, including myopathies and muscular dystrophies, for whom only 25% to 50%[5–8] receive a diagnosis after WES. RNA was sourced from 63 patients, 13 of whom had prior diagnoses with variants expected to influence transcription (such as loss-of-function or essential splice site variants), and 50 of whom were genetically undiagnosed. The undiagnosed cases included those for whom prior genetic analysis had prioritized variants predicted to alter RNA splicing or strong candidate genes, in addition to cases with no strong candidate from prior genetic analysis. RNA was isolated from muscle tissue biopsy, obtained routinely during the diagnostic evaluation of primary muscle disease patients.

Here, the study compared each patient with 184 control skeletal muscle samples available through the GTEx database,[63] an RNA-seq compendium of health donors across multiple tissues. For the detection of transcript-level changes, Z-scores were computed on the logarithm of gene length normalized read counts by subtracting the mean count and dividing by the standard deviation. Expression outliers were identified as those with an absolute Z-score of greater than 3, with no test of significance performed. The expression outlier analysis did not yield any convincing candidates. To identify rare splice events, outlier events were considered that were maximal in a given sample and less than half in the next highest sample. Their approach focused on identifying transcriptional aberrations in a defined list of neuromuscular disorder–associated genes.[22]

Using this approach RNA-seq (re)identified all putative disease-causing splice variants in the 13 diagnosed patients and, thus, validated the capability of this approach to identify transcriptional aberrations and enabling its use in the subsequent discovery of novel disease-causing variants in undiagnosed cases. The method results in a median of 5 potentially pathogenic splice events per samples in 190 neuromuscular disorder associated genes. Resulting in an overall diagnosis of 35% of the undiagnosed patients (17 of 50).[22] Remarkably, 4 of 17 of these cases harbored the same recurrent de novo intronic variant in COL6A1, resulting in a dominantly acting splice-gain aberration and 23 further cases were identified in an external collagen VI–like dystrophy cohort, explaining approximately 25% of cases with clinically suspected collagen VI dystrophy in whom prior genetic analysis is negative.

THE KEY ADVANTAGES OF RNA-SEQ

Newly diagnosed cases in these studies highlight the key advantages of RNA-seq in rare Mendelian disorder diagnosis (**Box 1**). In 4 patients with a rare muscle disorder harboring an extended splice site VUS, RNA-seq confirmed splice disruption in 2 patients with no observable effect on local splicing patterns in the remaining 2 patients, emphasizing the value of RNA-seq in ruling out nonpathogenic VUS. Remarkably, RNA-seq enabled pathogenicity to be assigned to a number of putatively benign synonymous variants. Cummings and colleagues detected a synonymous variant in

---

Box 1
Key Advantages of Transcriptome Sequencing in Mendelian Disorder Diagnosis

- Direct insight into the transcriptional perturbations of genetic variation.
- Identification of noncoding pathogenic variants unobservable by whole exome sequencing.
- Identification of noncoding pathogenic variants too abundant to be interpreted by whole genome sequencing.
- Reprioritization of variants of unknown significance detected by whole exome sequencing and whole genome sequencing.
- Resolving pathogenicity of noncoding and coding variants of unknown significance (including synonymous variants).
- Value in ruling out nonpathogenic variants of unknown significance.
- Identifying a practicable number of strong candidates for validation.
- Discovery of new disease-associated genes.
- Provision of genetic diagnoses for undiagnosed cases.

RYR1 resulting in an exonic splice gain owing to strengthening of a novel splice site over that of the canonical splice site and in *POMGNT1* resulting in exon skipping secondary to disruption of a splice motif. Notably, identification of aberrant splicing not only provided pathogenic confirmation of exonic variants, but also enabled the identification of pathogenic noncoding variants. Kremer and colleagues[21] described a homozygous deep intronic variant leading to a defective splice event (creation of a pseudoexon resulting in a premature stop codon) and subsequent loss of function in *TIMMDC1*. *TIMMDC1* also appeared as an expression outlier in the analysis, presumably owing to nonsense-mediated decay. Importantly, this study also revealed the occurrence of cryptic exons arising from loci with weak background splicing (approximately 1% in the general population), termed cryptic splice sites, in 2 patients, thus, providing a valuable clue for variant prioritization because rare variants in these locations are more likely to affect splicing.[21]

CHALLENGES IN RNA-SEQ APPROACHES
Disease-Relevant Tissue Selection

Both studies identified tissue selection as a considerable obstacle. It is natural to question whether RNA-seq analysis of unaffected tissues can reliably aid in genetic diagnosis, owing to the presumably negligible physiologic consequence of the variant in the tissue.[21] However, Mendelian disorders frequently show specificity to selected tissue(s) which are unobtainable for RNA-seq in a premortem setting, necessitating exploration of surrogate tissues.

Because gene expression and messenger RNA isoforms vary widely across tissues types[64,65], the identification of proxy tissues using the GTEx database, with careful consideration of expression status of the relevant genes, is one proposed way to circumnavigate the potentially underpowered analysis to detect relevant transcriptional aberrations in unaffected, easily accessible tissues.[22] Reprogramming of patient cells into induced pluripotent stem cells and differentiation into disease-relevant tissues may also be used in cases of high-interest or theoretic possibility, such as the recently published use of induced pluripotent stem cells and RNA-seq to pinpoint the noncoding disease-causing variant in *TAF1* responsible for X-linked dystonia–parkinsonism.[14]

In the case of mitochondrial disorders, patient fibroblast cell lines are a valuable surrogate for affected tissue, indicating that tissue specificity does not preclude RNA-seq of unaffected tissues. In fact, expression of 2574 of the 3768 disease genes (68%) listed in OMIM could be detected in fibroblast cell lines.[66] Moreover, nonaffected tissues have the advantage that the regulatory consequences on other genes are limited and, therefore, the causal defects are more likely be detected as outliers.[67] However, in the case of rare muscle disorders, poor expression of commonly disrupted muscle disorders genes in whole blood and fibroblasts necessitated biopsy of affected tissue for correct interpretation of genetic variation.[22]

Extensive Normalization and Statistical Assessments

Both studies highlight the need for closely matched, extensively normalized RNA-seq samples, requiring knowledge of technical variables, such as quality metrics (RNA integrity number), methodology (RNA extraction, library preparation), and phenotypic features, to exclude expression outliers from analysis, whether this be between patient samples[21] or with a database of public RNA-seq datasets such as GTEx.[22,63] Altogether, in this immature area, methods for detecting aberrant expression lack adequate assessment of statistical significance, use arbitrary cutoffs, and rely on manual correction for available confounders. A newly developed algorithm, OUTRIDER, addresses some of these issues (https://github.com/gagneurlab/OUTRIDER).

Future Prospects and Challenges for RNA-seq in Mendelian Disorder Diagnosis

The power of RNA-seq as a complementary tool to WES and WGS in identifying candidate variants for Mendelian disorders is clear. The flexibility and seemingly infinite methodologic and analytical options for RNA-seq present a double-edged sword, because these traits both spur discoveries while simultaneously complicating translation into the clinical diagnostic setting.[32] However, as with WES and WGS, which still uses multiple different platforms, protocols, and pipelines, we suspect that, given time and development of appropriate methodology, RNA-seq will establish itself in the clinical diagnostic pipeline for unsolved Mendelian disorders, given its increase in diagnostic yield, with blood as the likely easily accessible tissue of choice.

Multiomics Approaches and Data Sharing

With the ascension of multiomics approaches, encompassing genomics, epigenomics, transcriptomics, proteomics, and metabolomics, among others, there is an immense increase in the volume of exploitable data, giving rise to an increasingly integrated view of disease pathophysiology.[30] When these data are deposited into public databases, it becomes an invaluable resource for the broader scientific community, facilitating increase in study size and statistical power for more sophisticated data analyses.[68]

SUMMARY

The successful application of RNA-seq analysis in the setting of unsolved WES cases deems RNA-seq an essential companion to genome-based diagnostics, illustrated by the ability to validate suspected splice variants and the substantial increase in diagnostic yield. Integration of RNA-seq as a standardized diagnostic assay for all Mendelian disorders, akin to DNA sequencing, is within reach. To optimally investigate the true potential of RNA-seq in the diagnosis of Mendelian disorders and to establish the accuracy required for clinical translation, it is paramount that we collaborate on an international scale via the establishment of -omics data repositories.

REFERENCES

1. Ashley EA, Butte AJ, Wheeler MT, et al. Clinical assessment incorporating a personal genome. Lancet 2010;375(9725):1525–35.
2. Choi M, Scholl UI, Ji W, et al. Genetic diagnosis by whole exome capture and massively parallel DNA sequencing. Proc Natl Acad Sci U S A 2009;106(45): 19096–101.
3. Ng SB, Buckingham KJ, Lee C, et al. Exome sequencing identifies the cause of a Mendelian disorder. Nat Genet 2010;42(1):30.
4. Boycott KM, Rath A, Chong JX, et al. International cooperation to enable the diagnosis of all rare genetic diseases. Am J Hum Genet 2017;100(5):695–705.
5. Ankala A, da Silva C, Gualandi F, et al. A comprehensive genomic approach for neuromuscular diseases gives a high diagnostic yield. Ann Neurol 2015;77(2): 206–14.
6. Yang Y, Muzny DM, Xia F, et al. Molecular findings among patients referred for clinical whole-exome sequencing. JAMA 2014;312(18):1870–9.

7. Taylor JC, Martin HC, Lise S, et al. Factors influencing success of clinical genome sequencing across a broad spectrum of disorders. Nat Genet 2015;47(7):717.
8. Chong JX, Buckingham KJ, Jhangiani SN, et al. The genetic basis of Mendelian phenotypes: discoveries, challenges, and opportunities. Am J Hum Genet 2015; 97(2):199–215.
9. Bamshad MJ, Ng SB, Bigham AW, et al. Exome sequencing as a tool for Mendelian disease gene discovery. Nat Rev Genet 2011;12(11):745.
10. Wortmann SB, Koolen DA, Smeitink JA, et al. Whole exome sequencing of suspected mitochondrial patients in clinical practice. J Inherit Metab Dis 2015; 38(3):437–43.
11. Gilissen C, Hehir-Kwa JY, Thung DT, et al. Genome sequencing identifies major causes of severe intellectual disability. Nature 2014;511(7509):344.
12. Belkadi A, Bolze A, Itan Y, et al. Whole-genome sequencing is more powerful than whole-exome sequencing for detecting exome variants. Proc Natl Acad Sci U S A 2015;112(17):5473–8.
13. Stavropoulos DJ, Merico D, Jobling R, et al. Whole-genome sequencing expands diagnostic utility and improves clinical management in paediatric medicine. NPJ Genom Med 2016;1:15012.
14. Valente EM, Bhatia KP. Solving Mendelian mysteries: the non-coding genome may hold the key. Cell 2018;172(5):889–91.
15. Lionel AC, Costain G, Monfared N, et al. Improved diagnostic yield compared with targeted gene sequencing panels suggests a role for whole-genome sequencing as a first-tier genetic test. Genet Med 2018;20(4):435–43.
16. 1000 Genomes Project Consortium, Auton A, Brooks LD, Durbin RM, et al. A global reference for human genetic variation. Nature 2015;526(7571):68.
17. Sudmant PH, Rausch T, Gardner EJ, et al. An integrated map of structural variation in 2,504 human genomes. Nature 2015;526(7571):75.
18. MacArthur D, Manolio T, Dimmock D, et al. Guidelines for investigating causality of sequence variants in human disease. Nature 2014;508(7497):469.
19. Goldstein DB, Allen A, Keebler J, et al. Sequencing studies in human genetics: design and interpretation. Nat Rev Genet 2013;14(7):460.
20. Lek M, MacArthur D. The challenge of next generation sequencing in the context of neuromuscular diseases. J Neuromuscul Dis 2014;1(2):135–49.
21. Kremer LS, Bader DM, Mertes C, et al. Genetic diagnosis of Mendelian disorders via RNA sequencing. Nat Commun 2017;8:15824.
22. Cummings BB, Marshall JL, Tukiainen T, et al. Improving genetic diagnosis in Mendelian disease with transcriptome sequencing. Sci Transl Med 2017;9(386) [pii:eaal5209].
23. Jung H, Lee D, Lee J, et al. Intron retention is a widespread mechanism of tumor-suppressor inactivation. Nat Genet 2015;47(11):1242.
24. Li YI, van de Geijn B, Raj A, et al. RNA splicing is a primary link between genetic variation and disease. Science 2016;352(6285):600–4.
25. Cieślik M, Chinnaiyan AM. Cancer transcriptome profiling at the juncture of clinical translation. Nat Rev Genet 2018;19(2):93.
26. Sandmann S, De Graaf AO, Karimi M, et al. Evaluating variant calling tools for non-matched next-generation sequencing data. Sci Rep 2017;7:43169.
27. Eilbeck K, Quinlan A, Yandell M. Settling the score: variant prioritization and Mendelian disease. Nat Rev Genet 2017;18(10):599.
28. Cooper GM, Shendure J. Needles in stacks of needles: finding disease-causal variants in a wealth of genomic data. Nat Rev Genet 2011;12(9):628.

29. Karczewski KJ, Weisburd B, Thomas B, et al. The ExAC browser: displaying reference data information from over 60 000 exomes. Nucleic Acids Res 2016;45(D1): D840–5.
30. Lowe R, Shirley N, Bleackley M, et al. Transcriptomics technologies. PLoS Comput Biol 2017;13(5):e1005457.
31. Mortazavi A, Williams BA, McCue K, et al. Mapping and quantifying mammalian transcriptomes by RNA-seq. Nat Methods 2008;5(7):621.
32. Byron SA, Van Keuren-Jensen KR, Engelthaler DM, et al. Translating RNA sequencing into clinical diagnostics: opportunities and challenges. Nat Rev Genet 2016;17(5):257.
33. Adiconis X, Borges-Rivera D, Satija R, et al. Comparative analysis of RNA sequencing methods for degraded or low-input samples. Nat Methods 2013; 10(7):623.
34. TruSeq® RNA sample preparation v2 guide (Illumina). Available at: https:// support.illumina.com/content/dam/illumina-support/documents/documentation/ chemistry_documentation/samplepreps_truseq/truseqrna/truseq-rna-sample-prep-v2-guide-15026495-f.pdf.
35. Zhao S, Zhang Y, Gordon W, et al. Comparison of stranded and non-stranded RNA-seq transcriptome profiling and investigation of gene overlap. BMC Genomics 2015;16(1):675.
36. Levin JZ, Yassour M, Adiconis X, et al. Comprehensive comparative analysis of strand-specific RNA sequencing methods. Nat Methods 2010;7(9):709.
37. Wang Z, Gerstein M, Snyder M. RNA-seq: a revolutionary tool for transcriptomics. Nat Rev Genet 2009;10(1):57.
38. Eckersley-Maslin MA, Spector DL. Random monoallelic expression: regulating gene expression one allele at a time. Trends Genet 2014;30(6):237–44.
39. Reinius B, Sandberg R. Random monoallelic expression of autosomal genes: stochastic transcription and allele-level regulation. Nat Rev Genet 2015;16(11):653.
40. Lossie AC, Whitney MM, Amidon D, et al. Distinct phenotypes distinguish the molecular classes of Angelman syndrome. J Med Genet 2001;38(12):834–45.
41. Klimpe S, Zibat A, Zechner U, et al. Evaluating the effect of spastin splice mutations by quantitative allele specific expression assay. Eur J Neurol 2011;18(1): 99–105.
42. Wood DL, Nones K, Steptoe A, et al. Recommendations for accurate resolution of gene and isoform allele-specific expression in RNA-seq data. PLoS One 2015; 10(5):e0126911.
43. Rivas MA, Pirinen M, Conrad DF, et al. Human genomics. effect of predicted protein-truncating genetic variants on the human transcriptome. Science 2015; 348(6235):666–9.
44. Zhao J, Akinsanmi I, Arafat D, et al. A burden of rare variants associated with extremes of gene expression in human peripheral blood. Am J Hum Genet 2016; 98(2):299–309.
45. Tazi J, Bakkour N, Stamm S. Alternative splicing and disease. Biochim Biophys Acta 2009;1792(1):14–26.
46. Scotti MM, Swanson MS. RNA mis-splicing in disease. Nat Rev Genet 2016; 17(1):19.
47. Singh RK, Cooper TA. Pre-mRNA splicing in disease and therapeutics. Trends Mol Med 2012;18(8):472–82.
48. Soemedi R, Cygan KJ, Rhine CL, et al. Pathogenic variants that alter protein code often disrupt splicing. Nat Genet 2017;49(6):848.

49. Xiong HY, Alipanahi B, Lee LJ, et al. RNA splicing. the human splicing code reveals new insights into the genetic determinants of disease. Science 2015; 347(6218):1254806.
50. Harrow J, Frankish A, Gonzalez JM, et al. GENCODE: the reference human genome annotation for the ENCODE project. Genome Res 2012;22(9):1760–74.
51. Li YI, Knowles DA, Humphrey J, et al. LeafCutter: annotation-free quantification of RNA splicing. Nat Genet 2018;50(1):151.
52. Pervouchine DD, Knowles DG, Guigo R. Intron-centric estimation of alternative splicing from RNA-seq data. Bioinformatics 2012;29(2):273–4.
53. Taylor RW, Pyle A, Griffin H, et al. Use of whole-exome sequencing to determine the genetic basis of multiple mitochondrial respiratory chain complex deficiencies. JAMA 2014;312(1):68–77.
54. Ohtake A, Murayama K, Mori M, et al. Diagnosis and molecular basis of mitochondrial respiratory chain disorders: exome sequencing for disease gene identification. Biochim Biophys Acta 2014;1840(4):1355–9.
55. Kohda M, Tokuzawa Y, Kishita Y, et al. A comprehensive genomic analysis reveals the genetic landscape of mitochondrial respiratory chain complex deficiencies. PLoS Genet 2016;12(1):e1005679.
56. Pronicka E, Piekutowska-Abramczuk D, Ciara E, et al. New perspective in diagnostics of mitochondrial disorders: two years' experience with whole-exome sequencing at a national paediatric centre. J Transl Med 2016;14(1):174.
57. Elstner M, Andreoli C, Ahting U, et al. MitoP2: an integrative tool for the analysis of the mitochondrial proteome. Mol Biotechnol 2008;40(3):306–15.
58. Wortmann SB, Mayr JA, Nuoffer JM, et al. A guideline for the diagnosis of pediatric mitochondrial disease: the value of muscle and skin biopsies in the genetics era. Neuropediatrics 2017;48(04):309–14.
59. Gorman GS, Chinnery PF, DiMauro S, et al. Mitochondrial diseases. Nat Rev Dis Primers 2016;2:16080.
60. Haack TB, Kopajtich R, Freisinger P, et al. ELAC2 mutations cause a mitochondrial RNA processing defect associated with hypertrophic cardiomyopathy. Am J Hum Genet 2013;93(2):211–23.
61. Haack TB, Danhauser K, Haberberger B, et al. Exome sequencing identifies ACAD9 mutations as a cause of complex I deficiency. Nat Genet 2010;42(12):1131.
62. Love MI, Huber W, Anders S. Moderated estimation of fold change and dispersion for RNA-seq data with DESeq2. Genome Biol 2014;15(12):550.
63. GTEx Consortium. Human genomics. The genotype-tissue expression (GTEx) pilot analysis: multitissue gene regulation in humans. Science 2015;348(6235):648–60.
64. Mele M, Ferreira PG, Reverter F, et al. Human genomics. the human transcriptome across tissues and individuals. Science 2015;348(6235):660–5.
65. Wang ET, Sandberg R, Luo S, et al. Alternative isoform regulation in human tissue transcriptomes. Nature 2008;456(7221):470.
66. Kremer LS, Wortmann SB, Prokisch H. "Transcriptomics": molecular diagnosis of inborn errors of metabolism via RNA-sequencing. J Inherit Metab Dis 2018;41(3):525–32.
67. Gagneur J, Stegle O, Zhu C, et al. Genotype-environment interactions reveal causal pathways that mediate genetic effects on phenotype. PLoS Genet 2013;9(9):e1003803.
68. Sham PC, Purcell SM. Statistical power and significance testing in large-scale genetic studies. Nat Rev Genet 2014;15(5):335.

The Evolution of Constitutional Sequence Variant Interpretation

Jessica Mester, MS[a],*, Tina Pesaran, MS, MA[b]

KEYWORDS

- Variant classification • Genetic testing • Population data • Functional studies
- In silico • de novo • Quantitative • ACMG-AMP

KEY POINTS

- A combination of different types of evidence incorporating population data, functional studies, clinical data, and predictive tools is necessary for thorough, thoughtful variant classification.
- Variant classification criteria may be optimized in a quantitative, gene-specific manner using validated predictors of pathogenicity for genes or conditions with sufficient information.
- Large-scale data (genome sequencing of healthy and affected cohorts, high-throughput functional studies, and in silico metapredictors) increase the robustness of evidence used for variant classification and lend themselves to incorporation in quantitative frameworks.
- Collaborative efforts by laboratories and disease-specific expert groups reduce variant classification discrepancies and improve the quality of variant interpretation information available to patients and researchers.

INTRODUCTION

Sequence variants may be detected in an individual's germline DNA by molecular genetic testing performed in diagnostic, predictive, or preventive clinical settings. Interpretation of variants detected via this testing is complex and requires gathering multiple pieces of information to be analyzed in the context of the clinical presentation and the gene or disorder under consideration. This article reviews the history of

This article originally appeared in *Advances in Molecular Pathology*, Volume 2, 2019.
Disclosure: J. Mester is an employee of GeneDx, Inc., a wholly owned subsidiary of OPKO Health, Inc. T. Pesaran is an employee of Ambry Genetics, a wholly owned subsidiary of Konica-Minolta.
[a] GeneDx Inherited Cancer Program, Gaithersburg, MD, USA; [b] Variant Assessment Program, Ambry Genetics, 15 Argonaut, Aliso Viejo, CA 92656, USA
* Corresponding author. 1425 Grace Ave, Lakewood, OH 44107.
E-mail address: jmester@genedx.com

germline sequence variant interpretation, highlighting the lines of evidence used in current variant interpretation practices. It also considers how developments in sequencing and other technologies have provided data that have enhanced the ability to interpret genetic variants.

SIGNIFICANCE

Molecular germline genetic testing has evolved from a niche service consisting of single-gene testing for affected individuals exclusively by genetics providers, to multi-gene panels or exome testing for either affected or unaffected individuals offered by any clinician, and will one day involve routine genome sequencing of healthy individuals as a part of primary care preventive medical practice. Expanding the scope of genetic testing as well as the population undergoing analysis brings new challenges to analyzing results. Inaccurate variant interpretation can have dire consequences for patients. For genes associated with high cancer risks, detection of a variant deemed pathogenic can lead patients to make surgical decisions that are irreversible should the variant classification subsequently change based on new information. Specific medications or therapies to treat seizure disorders or metabolic conditions may be offered to or contraindicated for patients with pathogenic variants in specific genes. These factors drive the need for a careful, evidence-based approach to variant interpretation for individuals pursuing molecular genetic testing regardless of the clinical indication.

A BRIEF HISTORY OF SEQUENCE VARIANT INTERPRETATION

Clinical testing for sequence variants and copy number changes may be performed on an individual's germline DNA to diagnose a hereditary disorder based on clinical phenotype or family history, or may also be undertaken to screen healthy individuals for disease risk. This testing seeks to identify changes, or variants, in the patient's DNA that differ from a "healthy" reference sequence. Inevitably, the more genes that are analyzed, the more variants are bound to be detected. The challenge then becomes interpretation of these variants: gathering evidence to determine whether they should be considered pathogenic (disease causing) or benign (not associated with disease risk).

Although it may seem logical to assume that a truncating variant (one that disrupts the protein's reading frame, leading to its decay or removal of an essential functional domain) in a gene for which loss of function is the mechanism of disease would be pathogenic, this does not always hold true. For example, exons 26 and 32 of TSC2 (GenBank NM000548.3), also described as exons 25 and 31 using alternate exon numbering, are subject to alternative splicing, and truncating or frameshift variants in these regions have been identified in adults lacking features consistent with tuberous sclerosis complex.[1] Likewise, it can be tempting to consider a missense variant as pathogenic if it occurs in a functionally important protein domain, but subsequent functional studies may reveal no impact, or the variant may be present at high population frequency. It is therefore necessary to have gene-specific rules to guide the process of variant classification that take into account multiple lines of evidence and combine them to determine variant pathogenicity.

More than 20 years ago, Cotton and Scriver[2] suggested criteria for determining whether a DNA variant was phenotype-modifying or neutral, specifying type of variant, segregation studies, population frequency, and functional studies, along with the extent of DNA analysis performed, as helpful pieces of information for variant classification. These lines of evidence continued to serve as core criteria for other qualitative and quantitative gene-specific variant classification models.[3–7] However, one laboratory or expert group might place a higher or lower level of importance on the same piece of evidence, leading to discrepant classifications for the same variant, and to confusion for patients and providers.[8]

Major steps forward in harmonizing the approach to variant classification occurred with publications from the American College of Medical Genetics and Genomics (ACMG) in 2000[9] and 2008[10] and coauthored with the Association for Molecular Pathology (AMP) in 2015.[11] The 2015 ACMG/AMP guidelines outline a qualitative approach to variant classification incorporating data from several lines of evidence: population data, computational and predictive data, functional data, segregation data, de novo data, allelic data, phenotype specificity, co-occurrence data, and expert opinion. These guidelines have also been adopted by the UK-based Association for Clinical Genomic Science. Variant curation expert panels developed under the auspices of ClinGen (www.clinicalgenome.org) are using the ACMG/AMP guidelines as a framework, publishing modified versions of the guidelines tailored for gene-specific use. Of note, these guidelines were crafted for use in the classification of mendelian disorders, as opposed to more common and complex polygenic conditions or somatic cancer, and are relevant to sequence variants detected by Sanger, next-generation, or other sequencing methodologies as opposed to copy number variants. In addition, the ACMG/AMP guidelines provide guidance regarding the nomenclature used to define pathogenicity and likelihood for each category (**Fig. 1**).[12]

This article focuses on each line of evidence specified in the ACMG/AMP guidelines (**Fig. 2**), providing background regarding the utility of each criterion for sequence variant classification purposes. Readers are referred to the ACMG/AMP guidelines[11] for definitions regarding the proposed evidence codes (eg, PVS1, PM5, PP4) that are referred to in this article.

LINES OF EVIDENCE USED IN SEQUENCE VARIANT INTERPRETATION
Predicted Effect on Protein and Disease Mechanism

The first step in variant interpretation is to understand the nature of the gene-disease mechanism. Does the gene act via a loss-of-function (LoF) mechanism or a gain-of-function/dominant-negative effect? Protein-truncating variants, most of which lead to nonsense-mediated decay and haploinsufficiency, in genes with an LoF mechanism have a high prior probability of being pathogenic. This probability is captured in the ACMG/AMP rule code PVS1, which is considered to be very strong evidence supporting pathogenicity. PVS1 also encompasses other types of alterations that have a high probability of leading to haploinsufficiency, such those that affect the initiation site, canonical plus or minus 1 or 2 splice sites, certain intragenic tandem duplications, and single-exon or multiexon deletions. It may be inappropriate to apply a very strong evidence level toward pathogenicity for LoF variants in the following situations:

- The gene's mechanism of disease is not LoF
- The variant causes protein truncation but does not result in NMD

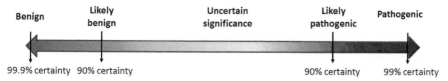

Fig. 1. Thresholds used for variant classification in the ACMG/AMP framework.

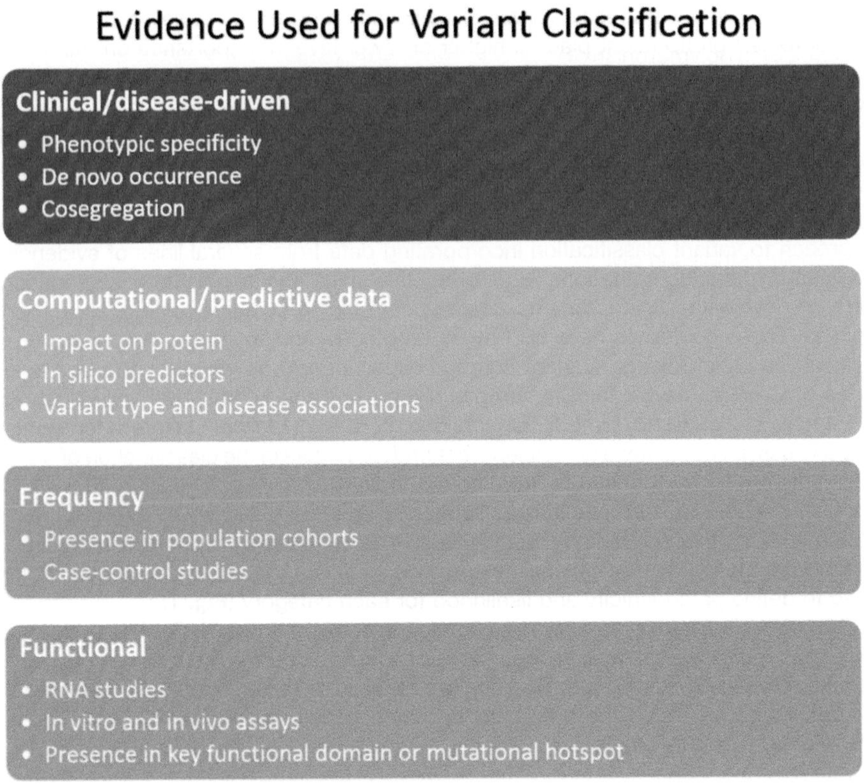

Evidence Used for Variant Classification

Clinical/disease-driven
- Phenotypic specificity
- De novo occurrence
- Cosegregation

Computational/predictive data
- Impact on protein
- In silico predictors
- Variant type and disease associations

Frequency
- Presence in population cohorts
- Case-control studies

Functional
- RNA studies
- In vitro and in vivo assays
- Presence in key functional domain or mutational hotspot

Fig. 2. Evidence incorporated into variant classification.

- The variant results in an in-frame deletion
- The variant occurs in a region that is subject to alternative splicing

However, the ACMG/AMP guidelines do not expand on how these caveats would affect use of the PVS1 code. Abou Tayoun and colleagues[13] provide a decision tree for modifying the strength of PVS1 that takes into account the type of variant, location within the protein, and other evidence.

Other ACMG/AMP criteria based on protein impact and knowledge regarding variant spectrum include:

- PP2: used to support a possible role in disease causation for a missense variant in a gene in which (1) missense variants are a common disease mechanism, and (2) benign missense variants are uncommon. BP1: used to support a benign role for a missense variant in a gene in which only truncating variants are known to cause disease.
- PM4: moderate pathogenic evidence for variants that change the length of the protein; this may include in-frame deletions or duplications or variants that extend protein length.
- BP3: supports a benign role for an in-frame deletion of a repetitive sequence in a region with no known function.
- BP7: supports a benign role for a synonymous (silent) variants not proved or predicted to affect splicing.

Population Data

Historically, a polymorphism was defined as an allele present in at least 1% of the general population.[14] Given their high frequency and the rare nature of most genetic disorders, it follows that variants present at high enough population frequency, to be defined as polymorphisms, would be considered harmless, with several notable exceptions (**Table 1**).

Early work to understand the diversity of alleles in global populations was limited by high sequencing cost, quality control limitations, and lack of sufficiently powered sequencing studies in diverse ancestral groups.[15,16] As the efficiency of sequencing technology has increased, genome-wide studies of larger, apparently healthy, or general population cohorts have allowed better understanding of the global allele diversity. In particular, gnomAD[17] (https://gnomad.broadinstitute.org/) includes exome sequencing data from more than 125,000 unrelated individuals and whole-genome sequencing for an additional 15,000 persons, with specific allele frequencies available for several subpopulations. Other databases focusing on specific subpopulations are listed in **Table 2**.

Population data may provide evidence leading to either a benign or pathogenic classification. A variant with population frequency greater than 5% can take a variant directly to benign through application of the ACMG/AMP stand-alone benign criterion BA1. Strong evidence toward a benign classification may also be achieved when a variant is present at a high enough allele frequency to be inconsistent with disease causation. No allele frequency threshold for BS1 (strong benign evidence) application was purposefully set so that cutoffs could be established in a disease-specific or gene-specific manner. Whiffin and colleagues[18] published a strategy to set disease-specific population frequency cutoffs taking into consideration condition prevalence, allelic and genetic heterogeneity, and disease penetrance, and created a freely available online calculator for maximum credible allele frequency calculation (https://cardiodb.org/allelefrequencyapp/). Absence of a variant within a large unaffected population cohort may hint at disease association, and is designated as moderate evidence toward pathogenicity by ACMG/AMP (PM2), although caution must be taken regarding this. Although the emergence of population-specific allele frequency data is vastly improved by resources such as gnomAD, not all populations are well represented. Thus, if the particular patient is from a population that may not have been captured in existing population resources, it remains possible that the variant in

Table 1
Examples of Pathogenic Sequence Variants at 1% or Higher Allele Frequency in Specific Populations

Gene and Variant	Disorder	Approximate Population Frequencies
CFTR c.1521_1523delCTT (p.Phe508del), commonly referred to as delta F508 (ΔF508) (NM_000492.3)	Cystic fibrosis	1 in 25 white people
HBB c.20A>T (p.Glu7Val) (NM_000518.5)	Sickle cell disease	1 in 10 African Americans
BRCA1 c.68_69delAG (p.Glu23Valfs) (NM_007294.3) *BRCA2* c.5946delT (p.Ser1982Argfs) (NM_000059.3)	Hereditary breast and ovarian cancer, Fanconi anemia	1 in 100 Ashkenazi Jews 1 in 62 Ashkenazi Jews
GJB2 c.109G>A (p.Val37Ile) (NM_004004.5)	Deafness	1 in 10 east Asians

Table 2
Ancestry-Specific Population Allele Frequency Databases

Database	Description	URL
The Greater Middle East Variome	Genome sequencing of 2497 Middle Eastern individuals	http://igm.ucsd.edu/gme/
Al Mena	Genomes and exome sequencing from 2115 Arab, Middle Eastern, and North African individuals	http://clingen.igib.res.in/almena/
Institute of Precision Medicine	Genome sequencing from 100 healthy volunteers and exome sequencing from 648 normal individuals; most persons of Singaporean Chinese ancestry	http://beacon.prism-genomics.org/
Korean Variant Archive	Exome sequencing of 1055 healthy Korean individuals	https://www.kobic.re.kr/kova/
Integrative Japanese Genome Variation	Genome sequencing of >3500 Japanese individuals	https://ijgvd.megabank.tohoku.ac.jp/

question is a benign finding endemic to the patient's ancestral group. In addition, rarity in and of itself may not be a specific predictor of pathogenicity.[19]

For highly penetrant conditions for which onset is expected before adulthood, identifying a variant in multiple unaffected individuals suggests a benign classification (ACMG/AMP BS2). However, the natural history of the disorder as well as the demographic features of the unaffected control population being studied are important considerations.

Functional Studies

Studying organisms and genes that have acquired changes in their nucleotide sequences is a fundamental practice in biology. In vivo or in vitro functional studies, assessing germline variant impact, is often an important aspect of making gene-disease associations and, once established, can be used in the classification of that alteration. For rare variants, robust, clinically validated functional studies are often the key to classification, especially when other lines of evidence, such as cosegregation or case-control data, are scarce.[20]

A well-established, statistically validated functional study can be weighted as a strong line of evidence for or against pathogenicity (PS3 and BS3, respectively). The ACMG/AMP guidelines recommend that, for a well-established study, the following be considered:

- The biological environment
- Whether the assay reflects the full spectrum of functions of the protein
- The validation, reproducibility, and robustness of the assay

Assays with high positive and negative predictive values that are reproducible and functionally appropriate can be weighted as strong evidence. However, it can be challenging to find studies that meet these criteria, and the ACMG/AMP guidelines do not provide guidance on what data are needed to deem an assay well established. After evaluating the evidence at hand, expert groups may decide to consider the body of functional evidence as strong if multiple studies replicate the same result. Alternatively, the weight of functional evidence could be decreased if appropriate functional studies are available but have not been statistically validated or replicated.[21]

To keep up with the increasing rates of variants identified by multigene panel testing, functional studies that are both high throughput and clinically validated will be of critical importance. An early example of large-scale functional analysis was published in 2003 by Kato and colleagues,[22] who used comprehensive site-directed mutagenesis in a yeast-based assay to evaluate all possible missense substitutions caused by single nucleotide variants throughout the p53 protein. As new technologies such as saturation mutagenesis are more widely used, multiplexed functional assays for large numbers of variants in single experiments will become more readily available.[23] Depending on the sensitivity and specificity of the assays, these could have a significant impact for variant classification, particularly for rare variants that lack other helpful evidence.

In Silico Predictors

In the absence of functional studies, computational in silico tools may provide a lower-confidence prediction as a proxy. These tools can be grouped into those that examine potential splicing defects and those that predict whether an amino acid change, mostly missense, is likely to damage the protein. Under the ACMG/AMP framework, in silico predictors are given the lowest level of evidence (supporting) when multiple predictors are in complete concordance. However, these guidelines do not specify how many predictors should be explored or which should be used, which can lead to variant classification discrepancies between clinical laboratories because using different predictors may increase the rates of variants classified as being of uncertain significance if 1 discordant prediction prevents application of the PP3 (pathogenic evidence) or BP4 (benign evidence) criteria.[24,25] Sun and Yu[26] found that the predictive accuracy increases until an optimal performance is reached using 2 or 3 tools, but that sensitivity began to decrease when additional models were incorporated.

Variants that cause splicing defects can occur in introns or exons, and they may disrupt the consensus splice site, alter splicing regulatory sequences such as exonic and intronic splice enhancers and silencers, activate a cryptic splice site, or create an entirely new alternate splice site. Computational splicing predictors based on a variety of algorithms, including position weighted matrix, neural network analysis, maximum entropy distributions, and other machine learning methods, have been developed to predict potential splice defects.[27] Most of the models are designed to predict changes in the strength of the splice sites for U2-type introns (GT-AG), which account for 99% of introns.[28] Although U12-type introns (AT-AC) are rare, clinicians should be careful not to use models designed for U2-type introns to predict U12-type splice sites.

Predicting the pathogenicity of missense variants relies on a combination of features including evolutionary conservation and structural and/or functional features of the amino acid change.[26,29] Each computational tool is based on different principles and has its own strengths and weaknesses,[30,31] but improved performance may be seen when complementary models are combined to create a metapredictor.[32,33] Given that different metapredictors may include some of the same individual predictors in their algorithms, selecting one that performs the best after testing on a set of validated pathogenic and benign variants is the preferred strategy compared with using results from several different metapredictors to avoid circularity. However, complete avoidance of circularity may be impossible, because predictors might have been trained on the variants or proteins currently under analysis, leading to overfitting.[34]

Phenotypic Specificity and Case-Control Studies

Identifying a rare variant in an individual with a phenotype highly specific to a rare disorder may provide evidence supporting pathogenicity, in line with the ACMG/AMP PP4 criteria. For disorders with genetic heterogeneity, it may be wise to ensure that, to the extent possible, other candidate genes have also been analyzed with no pathogenic variants identified. Targeted exome studies may be particularly helpful toward this goal.[35–37] The rarity of the variant is also an important consideration. If a variant is present at significant allele frequency in the general population, 1 (or more) affected individuals with the relevant phenotype will be found to harbor the variant based on chance alone.

Case-control evidence may apply when multiple affected individuals share the same variant. In order to warrant evidence toward pathogenicity, particularly for strong evidence as awarded by the ACMG/AMP PS4 criteria, cases and controls must include well-phenotyped populations; be well-matched with respect to age, gender, ancestry, and other potential confounding factors; and should include enough individuals (be sufficiently powered) to detect statistically significant odds ratios.[38] However, given the rare nature and allelic heterogeneity observed in most mendelian diseases, it is uncommon that a case-control study for a rare mendelian disorder is sufficiently powered. For this reason, the ACMG/AMP criteria allow for a relaxed use of the PS4 case-control criteria to count multiple unrelated probands showing phenotypic specificity with the same variant.

Cosegregation with Disease

Cosegregation of a variant with disease is a valuable quantitative data point used in assessing the pathogenicity of germline variants, particularly for rare mendelian disorders. This concept is similar to genetic linkage analysis in that likelihood ratios are derived similarly to logarithm of the odds scores in linkage, but specifically concerning the segregation of the variant and not a linked marker.[39] The seminal linkage models, developed from the 1950s through the 1980s,[40,41] are based on the degree of relationship of the probands and the genotype and disease status of the tested relatives. The derived likelihood ratio is also a function of an assumed penetrance that includes the risk of disease and can be stratified by age and/or sex as well as the frequency of the disease allele. Jarvik and Browning[42] proposed a simpler approach for use with qualitative frameworks such as the ACMG/AMP guidelines. Given that segregation supports linkage to the allele as opposed to a specific variant, the strength of evidence assigned for segregation data may be adjusted based on the number of genes associated with the disease and degree of certainty that all potential disease-causing variants were identified during the testing process.

De Novo Occurrence

Identification of de novo variants has been greatly accelerated by the emergence of exome and genome trio sequencing, in which concordant analysis of the affected proband along with both parents can identify genetic variants unique to the proband while concordantly excluding nonpaternity and/or nonmaternity, providing evidence supporting a strong pathogenic criterion (PS2) per ACMG/AMP.[43] Before the advent of trio testing as a means to confirm parentage, separate analyses, such as microsatellite marker studies, could prove parentage but may not have been pursued. A nonpaternity rate of 1.9% has been identified among men with high paternity confidence, and higher rates (some greater than 10%) have been reported in other studies.[39] Thus, the ACMG/AMP guidelines give a lower, moderate evidence strength (PM6) for an assumed de novo variant in the absence of studies confirming parentage.

Although de novo occurrence can be helpful evidence supporting pathogenicity, any newborns may have up to 100 de novo variants within their genomes, with 1 or 2 predicted to alter the coding sequence.[43,44] For genes with expansive coding sequences, de novo variation has a higher a priori risk of occurring by chance.[45] Thus, the requirement that the patient's phenotype be consistent with the disease caused by the gene in question is key to the appropriate application of de novo criteria. The ClinGen Sequence Variant Interpretation Working Group has crafted guidelines for tempering the strength of evidence applied for de novo occurrence when phenotype specificity is lacking or the disorder has high heterogeneity, or for increasing strength when multiple probands with de novo occurrence are identified (https://clinicalgenome.org/site/assets/files/3461/svi_proposal_for_de_novo_criteria_v1_0.pdf).

Additional Evidence

Other types of evidence that may play a role in variant classification include:

- Presence in a mutational hotspot functional domain: moderate pathogenic evidence may be considered if a variant occurs in a critical functional domain or region known to harbor multiple pathogenic missense variants without any benign variation, indicating functional importance (ACMG/AMP PM1).
- Allelic data: whether a second known pathogenic variant occurs on the same (in cis) or opposite (in trans) allele as the variant of interest. Use of this criterion depends on the inheritance and mechanism of disease.
  - For autosomal recessive disorders, a variant of interest appearing in trans with a known pathogenic variant supports pathogenicity (ACMG/AMP PM3).
  - For dominant conditions for which biallelic pathogenic variants are incompatible with life or cause a severe phenotype, finding a variant in trans with a known pathogenic variant supports a benign classification (ACMG/AMP BP2).
  - Variants in cis or with unknown phase require a thoughtful approach. A variant occurring in cis with a variant predicted to result in nonsense-mediated decay would not be expressed, or 2 missense variants occurring on the same allele may work synergistically. If phase is unknown, other observations of the same 2 rare variants together in multiple individuals suggests they are in cis; likewise, observations of each variant independent of the other, or co-occurring with other variants, suggest they are in trans.
- Co-occurrence with other pathogenic variants: observation of a variant in an individual harboring other pathogenic variants explaining the patient's phenotype is an evidence against pathogenicity (ACMG/AMP BP5). Caution should be exercised for phenotypes with significant heterogeneity (eg, breast cancer) because there are multiple reports of individuals with rare pathogenic variants in more than 1 breast cancer predisposition gene.[46,47]

PRESENT RELEVANCE AND FUTURE AVENUES TO CONSIDER OR TO INVESTIGATE
The Shift to Quantitative and Bayesian Approaches

This article outlines a primarily qualitative, categorical approach to variant assessment. This approach is purposefully general so that the ACMG/AMP criteria can be used for classification of variants in any mendelian disorder. For well-studied genes with validated functional studies, in silico models, and clinical correlates, it is possible to make gene-specific variant classification criteria using a quantitative approach.

Calls for variant interpretation to be driven by a quantitative, bayesian approach have echoed in the literature for more than a decade, when bayesian approaches began to be used to classify variants in cancer predisposition genes.[48–50] More recently, Tavtigian and colleagues[51] developed a bayesian framework that takes the current ACMG/AMP categories and shifts them from a qualitative to a quantitative structure (**Table 3**). Among the benefits of this system are the opportunity to combine pathogenic and benign criteria when determining classification, as well as permitting clinicians to more clearly recognize where on the spectrum of benign to pathogenic a variant of uncertain significance may be.

VARIANT CURATION OUTCOMES USING QUALITATIVE AND QUANTITATIVE APPROACHES

Variant 1: PTEN c.392C>T (p.Thr131Ile)

Germline pathogenic *PTEN* variants are causative for PTEN Hamartoma Tumor syndrome (PHTS), an autosomal dominant disorder causing increased risk for benign and malignant tumors as well as neurodevelopmental phenotypes. This missense variant was curated by the ClinGen PTEN Variant Curation Expert Panel[21] and classified as pathogenic based on the following data:

- Functional data: strong impact on phosphatase activity (PS3)
- Clinical data: multiple probands with presumed de novo occurrence (PM6_Strong) and phenotypes highly specific for PHTS (PS4_Moderate)
- Population data: variant absent or very rare in large population cohorts (PM2)
- Computational/predictive: *PTEN* shows missense constraint, and missense variants are a common mechanism of disease in PHTS (PP2)

Under the qualitative ACMG/AMP framework, this variant has 2 strong, 2 moderate, and 1 supporting pathogenic criteria, leading to a final classification of pathogenic. Using the bayesian framework proposed by Tavtigian and colleagues,[51] even starting with a low prior probability of 0.10 (generic prior proposed by investigators and reasonable for a missense variant), a combined odds of pathogenicity of 13,617.91 is achieved, leading to a posterior probability of 0.999, consistent with the pathogenic classification achieved by the qualitative method.

Variant 2: MYH7 c.5588G>A (p.Arg1863Gln)

Germline pathogenic variants in *MYH7* are associated with risk for cardiomyopathy. This missense variant was curated by the ClinGen Inherited Cardiomyopathy Variant Curation Expert Panel[52] and classified as being of uncertain significance based on the following data:

- Clinical data: variant identified in 2 individuals with cardiomyopathy (PS4_Supporting).
- Population data: variant absent or very rare in large population cohorts (PM2).
- Computational/predictive: in silico tools predict damaging effect (PP3).

Under the ACMG/AMP framework, this evidence results in classification of uncertain significance. However, under the bayesian framework, again using a prior probability of 0.10, the combined odds of pathogenicity equals 38.91, leading to a posterior probability of pathogenicity of 0.812. Although this still results in a final classification of uncertain significance, the quantitative method shows that the variant is approaching the threshold to be classified as likely pathogenic and has potential to be reclassified in that direction with minimal additional evidence.

ClinGen and Data Sharing

The Clinical Genome Resource (ClinGen, www.clinicalgenome.org), funded by the United States National Institutes of Health, is dedicated to improving the

Table 3
Odds of Pathogenicity for American College of Medical Genetics and Genomics/Association for Molecular Pathology Criteria

ACMG/AMP Criterion	Tavtigian et al,[51] Odds of Pathogenicity
Pathogenic: very strong	350.0
Pathogenic: strong	18.7
Pathogenic: moderate	4.33
Pathogenic: supporting	2.08
Benign: strong	0.05
Benign: supporting	0.48

Data from Tavtigian SV, Greenblatt MS, Harrison SM, et al. Modeling the ACMG/AMP variant classification guidelines as a Bayesian classification framework. Genet Med.2018;20(9):1054-60.

understanding of genomic variation for use in clinical care and research.[53] Under the auspices of ClinGen, expert panels including clinicians, researchers, and diagnostic laboratory representatives are being organized to tailor the ACMG/AMP criteria for gene-specific variant curation.[54] Collaborative efforts such as those driven by ClinGen will enhance data sharing efforts and increase the quality and consistency of variant classification efforts among participating groups.[55]

SUMMARY

As the improvements in technologies used for variant detection have increased rapidly, so have the quality and quantity of data points available for use during the variant classification process. The numbers and diversity of individuals in the general population exome and genome sequencing cohorts have expanded; high-throughput techniques have functionally interrogated variants before their observation in a single patient; trio-based and other familial testing strategies have enabled detection of de novo variants and provided segregation data helpful to the variant classification process. At the same time, relationships among disease-specific experts and clinical laboratories will continue to grow through involvement in efforts such as the ClinGen project, providing opportunities to share expertise and data with the ultimate goal to benefit patients.

REFERENCES

1. Ekong R, Nellist M, Hoogeveen-Westerveld M, et al. Variants within TSC2 Exons 25 and 31 are very unlikely to cause clinically diagnosable tuberous sclerosis. Hum Mutat 2016;37(4):364–70.
2. Cotton RG, Scriver CR. Proof of "disease causing" mutation. Hum Mutat 1998; 12(1):1–3.
3. Easton DF, Deffenbaugh AM, Pruss D, et al. A systematic genetic assessment of 1,433 sequence variants of unknown clinical significance in the BRCA1 and BRCA2 breast cancer-predisposition genes. Am J Hum Genet 2007;81(5): 873–83.
4. Miller PJ, Duraisamy S, Newell JA, et al. Classifying variants of CDKN2A using computational and laboratory studies. Hum Mutat 2011;32(8):900–11.
5. Sosnay PR, Siklosi KR, Van Goor F, et al. Defining the disease liability of variants in the cystic fibrosis transmembrane conductance regulator gene. Nat Genet 2013;45(10):1160–7.

6. Thompson BA, Spurdle AB, Plazzer J-P, et al. Application of a 5-tiered scheme for standardized classification of 2,360 unique mismatch repair gene variants in the InSiGHT locus-specific database. Nat Genet 2014;46(2):107–15.

7. Walsh R, Mazzarotto F, Whiffin N, et al. Quantitative approaches to variant classification increase the yield and precision of genetic testing in Mendelian diseases: the case of hypertrophic cardiomyopathy. Genome Med 2019;11(1):5.

8. Harrison SM, Dolinsky JS, Knight Johnson AE, et al. Clinical laboratories collaborate to resolve differences in variant interpretations submitted to ClinVar. Genet Med 2017;19(10):1096–104.

9. ACMG recommendations for standards for interpretation of sequence variations. Genet Med 2000;2:302.

10. Richards CS, Bale S, Bellissimo DB, et al. ACMG recommendations for standards for interpretation and reporting of sequence variations: Revisions 2007. Genet Med 2008;10(4):294–300.

11. Richards S, Aziz N, Bale S, et al. Standards and guidelines for the interpretation of sequence variants: a joint consensus recommendation of the American College of Medical Genetics and Genomics and the Association for Molecular Pathology. Genet Med 2015;17(5):405–24.

12. Plon SE, Eccles DM, Easton D, et al. Sequence variant classification and reporting: recommendations for improving the interpretation of cancer susceptibility genetic test results. Hum Mutat 2008;29(11):1282–91.

13. Abou Tayoun AN, Pesaran T, DiStefano MT, et al. Recommendations for interpreting the loss of function PVS1 ACMG/AMP variant criterion. Hum Mutat 2018; 39(11):1517–24.

14. Brookes AJ. The essence of SNPs. Gene 1999;234(2):177–86.

15. International HapMap 3 Consortium, Altshuler DM, Gibbs RA, et al. Integrating common and rare genetic variation in diverse human populations. Nature 2010; 467(7311):52–8.

16. 1000 Genomes Project Consortium, Auton A, Brooks LD, Durbin RM, et al. A global reference for human genetic variation. Nature 2015;526(7571):68–74.

17. Lek M, Karczewski KJ, Minikel EV, et al. Analysis of protein-coding genetic variation in 60,706 humans. Nature 2016;536(7616):285–91.

18. Whiffin N, Minikel E, Walsh R, et al. Using high-resolution variant frequencies to empower clinical genome interpretation. Genet Med 2017;19(10):1151–8.

19. Young EL, Feng BJ, Stark AW, et al. Multigene testing of moderate-risk genes: be mindful of the missense. J Med Genet 2016;53(6):366–76.

20. Brnich SE, Rivera-Muñoz EA, Berg JS. Quantifying the potential of functional evidence to reclassify variants of uncertain significance in the categorical and Bayesian interpretation frameworks. Hum Mutat 2018;39(11):1531–41.

21. Mester JL, Ghosh R, Pesaran T, et al. Gene-specific criteria for PTEN variant curation: recommendations from the ClinGen PTEN expert panel. Hum Mutat 2018; 39(11):1581–92.

22. Kato S, Han S-Y, Liu W, et al. Understanding the function-structure and function-mutation relationships of p53 tumor suppressor protein by high-resolution missense mutation analysis. Proc Natl Acad Sci U S A 2003;100(14):8424–9.

23. Gasperini M, Starita L, Shendure J. The power of multiplexed functional analysis of genetic variants. Nat Protoc 2016;11(10):1782–7.

24. Maxwell KN, Hart SN, Vijai J, et al. Evaluation of ACMG-guideline-based variant classification of cancer susceptibility and non-cancer-associated genes in families affected by breast cancer. Am J Hum Genet 2016;98(5):801–17.

25. Ghosh R, Oak N, Plon SE. Evaluation of in silico algorithms for use with ACMG/AMP clinical variant interpretation guidelines. Genome Biol 2017;18(1):225.

26. Sun H, Yu G. New insights into the pathogenicity of non-synonymous variants through multi-level analysis. Sci Rep 2019;9(1):1667.

27. Moles-Fernández A, Duran-Lozano L, Montalban G, et al. Computational tools for splicing defect prediction in breast/ovarian cancer genes: how efficient are they at predicting RNA alterations? Front Genet 2018;9:366.

28. Sibley CR, Blazquez L, Ule J. Lessons from non-canonical splicing. Nat Rev Genet 2016;17(7):407–21.

29. Katsonis P, Koire A, Wilson SJ, et al. Single nucleotide variations: biological impact and theoretical interpretation. Protein Sci 2014;23(12):1650–66.

30. Tavtigian SV, Greenblatt MS, Lesueur F, et al, IARC Unclassified Genetic Variants Working Group. In silico analysis of missense substitutions using sequence-alignment based methods. Hum Mutat 2008;29(11):1327–36.

31. Jordan DM, Ramensky VE, Sunyaev SR. Human allelic variation: perspective from protein function, structure, and evolution. Curr Opin Struct Biol 2010;20(3):342–50.

32. Ioannidis NM, Rothstein JH, Pejaver V, et al. REVEL: an ensemble method for predicting the pathogenicity of rare missense variants. Am J Hum Genet 2016;99(4):877–85.

33. Hart SN, Hoskin T, Shimelis H, et al. Comprehensive annotation of BRCA1 and BRCA2 missense variants by functionally validated sequence-based computational prediction models. Genet Med 2019;21(1):71–80.

34. Grimm DG, Azencott C-A, Aicheler F, et al. The evaluation of tools used to predict the impact of missense variants is hindered by two types of circularity. Hum Mutat 2015;36(5):513–23.

35. Polla DL, Cardoso MTO, Silva MCB, et al. Use of targeted exome sequencing for molecular diagnosis of skeletal disorders. PLoS One 2015;10(9):e0138314.

36. Weinberg CR, Umbach DM. Choosing a retrospective design to assess joint genetic and environmental contributions to risk. Am J Epidemiol 2000;152(3):197–203.

37. Campbell H, Rudan I. Interpretation of genetic association studies in complex disease. Pharmacogenomics J 2002;2(6):349–60.

38. Anderson KG. How well does paternity confidence match actual paternity?: Evidence from worldwide nonpaternity rates. Curr Anthropol 2006;47(3):513–20.

39. Goldgar DE. Collection and analysis of pedigree data. Birth Defects Orig Artic Ser 1984;20(6):61–76.

40. Morton NE. Sequential tests for the detection of linkage. Am J Hum Genet 1955;7(3):277–318.

41. Lalouel JM, Morton NE. Complex segregation analysis with pointers. Hum Hered 1981;31(5):312–21.

42. Jarvik GP, Browning BL. Consideration of cosegregation in the pathogenicity classification of genomic variants. Am J Hum Genet 2016;98(6):1077–81.

43. Ku CS, Polychronakos C, Tan EK, et al. A new paradigm emerges from the study of de novo mutations in the context of neurodevelopmental disease. Mol Psychiatry 2013;18(2):141–53.

44. Acuna-Hidalgo R, Veltman JA, Hoischen A. New insights into the generation and role of de novo mutations in health and disease. Genome Biol 2016;17(1):241.

45. MacArthur DG, Manolio TA, Dimmock DP, et al. Guidelines for investigating causality of sequence variants in human disease. Nature 2014;508(7497):469–76.

46. Couch FJ, Shimelis H, Hu C, et al. Associations between cancer predisposition testing panel genes and breast cancer. JAMA Oncol 2017;3(9):1190–6.

47. Frey MK, Sandler G, Sobolev R, et al. Multigene panels in Ashkenazi Jewish patients yield high rates of actionable mutations in multiple non-BRCA cancer-associated genes. Gynecol Oncol 2017;146(1):123–8.

48. Goldgar DE, Easton DF, Byrnes GB, et al. Genetic evidence and integration of various data sources for classifying uncertain variants into a single model. Hum Mutat 2008;29(11):1265–72.

49. Tavtigian SV, Greenblatt MS, Goldgar DE, et al, IARC Unclassified Genetic Variants Working Group. Assessing pathogenicity: overview of results from the IARC Unclassified Genetic Variants Working Group. Hum Mutat 2008;29(11): 1261–4.

50. Goldgar DE, Easton DF, Deffenbaugh AM, et al. Integrated evaluation of DNA sequence variants of unknown clinical significance: application to BRCA1 and BRCA2. Am J Hum Genet 2004;75(4):535–44.

51. Tavtigian SV, Greenblatt MS, Harrison SM, et al. Modeling the ACMG/AMP variant classification guidelines as a Bayesian classification framework. Genet Med 2018;20(9):1054–60.

52. Kelly MA, Caleshu C, Morales A, et al. Adaptation and validation of the ACMG/AMP variant classification framework for MYH7-associated inherited cardiomyopathies: recommendations by ClinGen's Inherited Cardiomyopathy Expert Panel. Genet Med 2018. https://doi.org/10.1038/gim.2017.218.

53. Rehm HL, Berg JS, Brooks LD, et al. ClinGen–the clinical genome resource. N Engl J Med 2015;372(23):2235–42.

54. Rivera-Muñoz EA, Milko LV, Harrison SM, et al. ClinGen Variant Curation Expert Panel experiences and standardized processes for disease and gene-level specification of the ACMG/AMP guidelines for sequence variant interpretation. Hum Mutat 2018;39(11):1614–22.

55. Harrison SM, Dolinksy JS, Chen W, et al. Scaling resolution of variant classification differences in ClinVar between 41 clinical laboratories through an outlier approach. Hum Mutat 2018;39(11):1641–9.

Clinical Bioinformatics in Precise Diagnosis of Mitochondrial Disease

Lishuang Shen, PhD[a], Elizabeth M. McCormick, MS, LCGC[b],
Colleen Clarke Muraresku, MS, LCGC[b], Marni J. Falk, MD[c],
Xiaowu Gai, PhD[a],*

KEYWORDS

- Clinical sequencing • Mitochondrial disease • Bioinformatics • Phenotype
- Pathogenicity • Variant annotation

KEY POINTS

- Sequencing-based genetic diagnosis of mitochondrial diseases faces extra special challenges owing to the involvement of mitochondrial DNA genome in disease etiology.
- In silico prediction of mitochondrial DNA variant effects needs specialized tools distinct from the tools developed for nuclear DNA variant annotation.
- Heteroplasmy and haplogroup are 2 key unique factors in interpreting the mitochondrial DNA variant effects for disease pathogenesis.
- MSeqDR, MitoMap, and HmtDB are among the major resources for mitochondrial disease and mitochondrial DNA genomics studies.

CLINICAL BIOINFORMATICS AND PRECISION MEDICINE

Precision medicine starts with a precise diagnosis. In contrast, clinical bioinformatics focuses on managing, analyzing, processing, and visualizing clinical and genomic data in a highly integrated manner. Clinical bioinformatics is therefore critically important for a genomics-based clinical diagnostic laboratory, which is a highly regulated environment. The primary type of data that clinical bioinformatics is concerned about in the diagnostic setting is the genotype data. Clinical bioinformaticians maintain and

[a] Keck School of Medicine of USC, Center for Personalized Medicine, Children's Hospital Los Angeles, Suite 300, 2100 West 3rd Street, Los Angeles, CA 90057, USA; [b] Mitochondrial Medicine Frontier Program, Children's Hospital of Philadelphia, 3401 Civic Center Boulevard, Philadelphia, PA 19104, USA; [c] CHOP Mitochondrial Medicine Frontier Program, Division of Human Genetics, Department of Pediatrics, University of Pennsylvania Perelman School of Medicine, The Children's Hospital of Philadelphia, ARC 1002c, 3615 Civic Center Boulevard, Philadelphia, PA 19104, USA
* Corresponding author.
E-mail address: xgai@chla.usc.edu

Clin Lab Med 40 (2020) 149–161
https://doi.org/10.1016/j.cll.2020.02.002
0272-2712/20/© 2020 Elsevier Inc. All rights reserved.
labmed.theclinics.com

develop information management systems to process the raw array and next-generation sequencing (NGS) data, and set up and operate analytical pipelines that distill the raw data into information and results, based on the clinical or phenotypic data, that are comprehensible to the medical directors for diagnostic reporting. The NGS data processing includes base calling and quality control (primary data analysis), alignment and variant calling (secondary analysis), and variant annotation and filtering (tertiary analysis). In the clinical diagnosis setting, the informatics system and processing pipelines must collect, validate, and monitor performance and quality control metrics according to standard operation procedures, in order to achieve regulatory certifications, such as College of American Pathologists.[1]

Another primary data type in clinical bioinformatics is clinical or phenotypic data. Genomic data analysis and interpretation has to be driven by the clinical phenotypes and is achieved through deep variant annotation, comprehensive and standardized clinical phenotype data representation, and phenotype-driven variant prioritization and interpretation. A comprehensive bioinformatics infrastructure is required to track patient samples from patient intake, sample accession, genomic data analysis, and all the way through clinical report generation and delivery.

NGS-based clinical diagnosis laboratories and companies have increased dramatically in recent years with the emergence and growing impacts of precision medicine. Major NGS-based clinical assays include especially molecular diagnostic and prognostic tests of rare Mendelian disorder, and both adult and pediatric cancers. Primary technologies applied in these assays include whole exome sequencing (WES), targeted panel sequencing, RNA-seq, and whole genome sequencing (WGS). The standard NGS data processing protocols, from raw reads to quality-filtered variant lists, have been largely well-established. We briefly introduce them here. We describe in greater depth the more individualized components of clinical bioinformatics in the diagnostic laboratories: clinical phenotype capturing and manipulation, along with phenotype-driven variant prioritization and interpretation for diagnostic reporting. We use mitochondrial diseases as an example of genetic disease diagnosis using NGS technologies and clinical bioinformatics.

Precise diagnosis in genomic medicine is a personalized diagnosis that identifies the casual relation between a patient's clinical phenotype profile and the genomic profile at the genome level, including both the nuclear and the mitochondrial genomes. For mitochondrial disease patients, the mitochondrial DNA (mtDNA) variant heteroplasmy levels also play a role in the precise diagnosis, as the same mtDNA variant might cause different diseases at different heteroplasmy levels.[2,3] In a prognostic and therapeutic sense, precise diagnosis guides proper treatments based on drug responses predicted from patient's clinical and genomic profiles.

MITOCHONDRIAL DISEASES AND SEQUENCING-BASED GENETIC DIAGNOSIS

Mitochondrial diseases are a clinically heterogeneous group of genetic disorders that are characterized by dysfunctional mitochondria. Mitochondrial diseases can occur at any age, and involve any organ or tissue in isolation, or, more frequently, involve multiple systems, typically affecting organs with high energy demands.[4]

The pathophysiology of mitochondrial diseases is complex and might be caused by genetic variants in either the mtDNA genome that encodes 13 structural peptide subunits of the oxidative phosphorylation system and 24 RNA molecules that are required for intramitochondrial protein synthesis, or the nuclear DNA (nDNA) genome, which encodes more than 1500 proteins that maybe required for healthy mitochondrial function, or the interplays between the mtDNA and nDNA variants.

Mitochondrial diseases can have any pattern of inheritance, including autosomal and X-linked inheritance for nDNA pathogenic variants and maternal inheritance for mtDNA pathogenic variants. In patients with pathogenic mtDNA variants, inheritance and clinical presentation are further complicated by the heteroplasmy,[3] and by the haplogroup background.[5,6] The heterogeneity in the genetic etiology and the clinical manifestations of mitochondrial diseases means that both diagnosis and management of these disorders are extremely difficult. Definitive diagnosis often depends on genetic testing, in addition to the histochemical and biochemical analysis of tissue biopsies. Determining the molecular etiology of primary mitochondrial disease in an affected individual can be particularly challenging given the extensive heterogeneity of clinical symptoms, poorly understood genotype–phenotype correlations, and nonspecific nature of many symptoms with significant clinical overlap for other conditions.[4,7]

Traditionally, the suspicious mitochondrial disease patients go through multiple biochemical and histochemical examinations, such as blood and cerebrospinal fluid testing for lactate and other metabolites for abnormality, MRI neuroimaging, and occasionally followed with candidate gene sequencing if clear clinical profile points to the genes. The poor clinical symptom–disease correlation in mitochondrial diseases and the limited coverage of candidate genes make this strategy less than ideal. So now the clinical diagnosis practice shifted to the more comprehensive NGS-based whole mtDNA genome, high-coverage panel (eg, MitoExome), WES, or RNA-seq sequencing (**Fig. 1**).

Whole Mitochondrial DNA Genome Sequencing

Many mitochondrial disease diagnostic companies or clinical centers offer sequencing of the whole mtDNA genome first, to obtain the diagnosis directly in a small percentage of cases or to exclude mitochondrial variants before performing WES or WGS mostly. This strategy allows for the identification of potentially pathogenic mtDNA variants and the accurate assessment of heteroplasmy levels. It is important to remember that the relevance of detecting many pathogenic mtDNA variants is restricted to clinically affected tissues such as skeletal muscle. Owing to technological progress, whole mtDNA genome coverage can often be obtained through WES or large-panel sequencing with an mtDNA augmentation protocol.[8]

Targeted Gene Panels

The panels with success in identifying pathogenic variants for mitochondrial diseases range from smaller focused gene panels to large panels targeting hundreds of the respiratory chain components and known disease-associated genes, and to the expansive "MitoExome" panel, which included all the 1100 genes listed in the MitoCarta inventory.[9–11] As comprehensive as MitoExome is, dozens of new mitochondrial disease genes not included in MitoExome have been found since its initial launch, which argues for the importance of an unbiased approach, such as WES.

Comprehensive, Unbiased, and Gene Agnostic Approaches (Whole Exome Sequencing, RNA-Seq, and Whole Genome Sequencing)

WES has revolutionized the molecular diagnosis of Mendelian mitochondrial diseases with success rate of detecting pathogenic variants in more than 50% patients.[12,13] Additionally, wide adaption of WES for mitochondrial diseases is the key contributor in identifying novel disease genes, which has pushed the total established mitochondrial disease genes to more than 300.[14] NGS-based molecular diagnosis is often less invasive than traditional biochemical strategies by avoiding the requirement for skin or

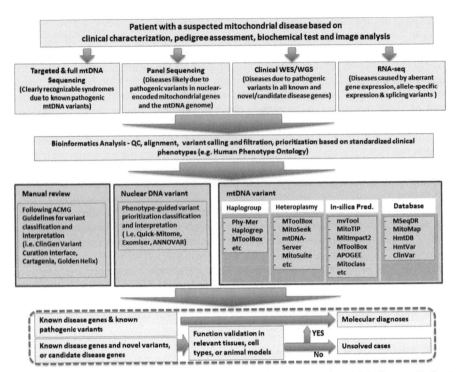

Fig. 1. Typical clinical sequencing workflow applicable to mitochondrial disease. Patient with a suspected mitochondrial disease is recommended to undergo a choice of different clinical sequencing strategy based on clinical characterization and pedigree assessment results. Standard bioinformatics analysis includes sequencing data quality control, alignment, variant calling and filtration, prioritization. Nuclear DNA variants undergo phenotype-guided prioritization classification and interpretation, whereas mitochondrial DNA (mtDNA) variants need heteroplasmy, haplogroup analysis and in silico and database annotations using mtDNA-specific tools. Finally, know pathogenic variants, or novel variants that can be validated by functional studies, are reported in molecular diagnosis following the American College of Medical Genetics guidelines for variant classification and interpretation. ACMG, American College of Medical Genetics.

muscle biopsies and, more important, has achieved much higher diagnosis rate than the approximately 11% found in conventional targeted Sanger sequencing.[15] The success of these studies has resulted in the accredited use of WES as not only a routine diagnostic tool, but also as the recommended first tier in clinical diagnostics.[13] WES in mitochondrial diseases may often results in most likely disease-causing variants being detected by could only be reported as a variant of unknown significance because they are not reported as known in reference databases like ClinVar or HGMD. The gene and variant curation efforts by teams like the Mitochondrial Disease Sequence Data Resource (MSeqDR) Consortium can help to identify new published pathogenic variants quicker than the generic resources like ClinVar, thus decreasing the likelihood of likely pathogenic and pathogenic variants being reported as a variant of unknown significance for mitochondrial diseases.

WES captures only the coding regions of the genome; thus, the disease-causing variants in noncoding regions such as splicing and regulatory regions may be missed, which is a concern for mitochondrial diseases RNA-seq can identify potential pathogenic aberrant splicing events, expression outliers, monoallelic expression.[16,17] In a systematic study that assessed a cohort of patients with unsolved primary muscle disorders, RNA-seq of patient-derived muscle achieved a diagnostic yield of 35% (17/50).[17]

WGS can detect variants in both the coding and noncoding regions, and thus has the potential to increase diagnostic yield in mitochondrial disease and other Mendelian diseases.[18] The barriers in WGS use for clinical diagnosis are (1) the higher sequencing laboratory cost and, more important, the analytical cost and resistance in reimbursement by health insurance company, and (2) the number of variants is large, typically more than 4 millions per genome. So there need to be more powerful tools for variant prioritization, adding the complexity of pathogenicity prediction and prioritization tools, and the lack of reference databases for noncoding region variants.

MITOCHONDRIAL DNA DATABASES AND MITOCHONDRIAL DISEASE DATABASES

Unlike the nDNA genome variants, the population reference databases for mtDNA variants have been falling behind until now. Major reference databases like gnoMAD, 1000 Genomes, and TopMED have not been providing the mtDNA data until recently, despite the abundant availability of WGS and WES data. The mtDNA genome specific databases include MitoMap[19] (https://www.mitomap.org/foswiki/bin/view/MITOMAP/WebHome), HmtDB[20,21] (https://www.hmtdb.uniba.it/), MSeqDR[22,23] (https://mseqdr.org), and a number of smaller databases. Except for the actively maintained MitoMap, MSeqDR, and HmtDB, most of the resources are not up to date, or are limited in their scope, features, and functions. MitoMap is a community resource database that has been recognized as the most authoritative for decades, providing an expertly curated and actively updated list of mtDNA variants and pathogenicity assessments, along with literature evidence. HmtDB is rich in data from in silico analysis, including the variability scores and transfer RNA (tRNA) variant effect predictions, along with recently added and enhanced HmtVar search and report tools. MitoMap and HmtDB both compile and report mtDNA variant allele frequency data derived from about 50,000 full-length mtDNA sequences deposited at GenBank that are largely overlapping.

MSeqDR constructs a large metapopulation reference for mtDNA variant allele frequencies, which provides position-specific variant information for up to 93,000 people at some positions. Of these, MSeqDR shares from MitoMap the synchronized approximately 50,000 full mtDNA genomes. In addition, MSeqDR mines data sources from literature and sequencing initiatives to add mtDNA variant data from more than 40,000 individuals. It is enhanced in particular with data from multiple Asian and other minority populations to achieve more comprehensive ethnic representations. Among them are the Sardinians population,[24] the Japanese population[25] (https://jmorp.megabank.tohoku.ac.jp), the aggregate data from 6391 individuals from GeneDx Inc.,[23] and 23,000 individuals from Kaviar.[26] We expect more comprehensive mtDNA allele frequency reference data from sequencing centers and molecular diagnosis companies in the future.

IN SILICO PREDICTION OF MITOCHONDRIAL DNA VARIANT EFFECTS

In silico prediction algorithms commonly used for nDNA variant assessment include Polyphen-2, SIFT, CADD score, Mutpred, and PROVEAN and were benchmarked extensively.[27] An evaluation of in silico algorithms for use with American College of Medical Genetics/Association of Molecular Pathology clinical variant interpretation guidelines ranked the newer metapredictors REVEL, MetaSVM, MetaLR, and VEST3 as top performers[27] over these long-standing algorithms, and recommended clinical laboratories to review and potentially update the algorithms currently in use in classification pipelines. These tools can be used in the molecular diagnosis of mitochondrial diseases when nDNA genes and variants are suspected. These algorithms, however, have shown poor accuracy when used for mtDNA variant pathogenicity assessment, as benchmarked on the manually curated mtDNA variants in MITOMAP and HmtVar.[28,29] According to the performance assessment of a set of 19 different prediction tools gathered in MitImpact2,[29] single criteria missense pathogenicity predictor tools for protein-coding variants performed the worst. Therefore, these tools are not recommended for direct application in mtDNA variant assessment.

To overcome the limitations of these single criteria predictors, ensemble tools were developed for mtDNA variants and some showed higher sensitivity and specificity in classifying pathogenic variants. One metapredictors tool MToolBox[30] calculates the composite Disease Score Estimation for nonsynonymous variants and tRNA variant based on structural, conservation, population data, in silico predictions, heteroplasmy, known pathogenicity status, and the functional evidences. APOGEE[31] and Mitoclass[32] are metapredictors tools for variants in protein-coding genes using machine learning based approaches. They are the multifactorial score tools that consider features including evolutionary conservation, primary, secondary or tertiary structure information, and functional and biochemical assays. MitImpact provides a precomputed collection of pathogenicity predictions for all nucleotide changes that cause nonsynonymous substitutions in human mitochondrial protein-coding genes.[29]

For mitochondrial tRNA variants, the Mitochondrial tRNA Informatics Predictor,[33] MToolBox, and PON-mt-RNA[34] (http://structure.bmc.lu.se/PON-mt-tRNA/datasets.html/) are the more commonly used. The Mitochondrial tRNA Informatics Predictor uses databases of pathogenic and benign variants, alignments between tRNAs of diverse species, structural information, and comparative genomics of tRNA mutation at positions in a generic tRNA to predict the impact of all possible single-base tRNA variants and deletions. These information sources were combined to provide a variant history and conservation score, position score of mutations at positions in a generic tRNA, and evaluated the steric impact of variants within any of the tRNA stems as secondary structure score. These 3 subscores are summarized to calculate the total pathogenicity score for each possible variant. Using a single point pathogenicity score cutoff, the system had sensitivity and specificity of 74%, better than PON-o-mt. The Mitochondrial tRNA Informatics Predictor provides downloadable collection of precomputed tRNA variant predictions for all nucleotide changes in tRNA coding genes. For rRNA variants, the heterologous inferential analysis[35,36] that is optimized for the mtDNA can be considered when assessing mtDNA variant pathogenicity.

HETEROPLASMY AND THE THRESHOLD EFFECT OF MITOCHONDRIAL DNA VARIANTS

Heteroplasmy is a unique phenomenon of mtDNA variants, relative to nDNA variants. Each cell can have many copies of mitochondria, and each mitochondrion in a cell can have multiple copies of the mtDNA genome. Heteroplasmy caused by different copies of mtDNA genomes carrying different alleles thus shows as a mixture of wild-type and variant alleles.[3] Owing to random segregation of mitochondria during cellular division, heteroplasmy levels may differ between tissues in a given individual. Heteroplasmy plays a pivotal role in the etiology of mitochondrial diseases, because most pathogenic mtDNA variants tend to be heteroplasmic in nature.[37] Some symptoms only manifest when the heteroplasmy reaches certain thresholds in specific tissues. Typically, the heteroplasmic threshold commonly quoted for many variants is in the 60% to

80% range in a given tissue for it to cause severe clinical symptoms.[6] Making things more complicated, such dependence on heteroplasmy levels varies in disease-specific and tissue-specific manors. The pathogenic tRNA[Leu] (UUR) m.3243A>G mutation is the best example of a heteroplasmy effect.[38] It causes different clinical phenotypes depending on the heteroplasmy levels. At 20% to 30% m.3243A>G mutant, patients commonly present with type 1 or type 2 diabetes or manifest autism. At 50% to 80% mutant, patients present with the mitochondrial myopathy, encephalopathy, lactic acidosis, and stroke syndrome. At 90% to 100% mutant, individuals manifest diseases such as Leigh syndrome. Cybrid studies proved that the changes in mtDNA heteroplasmy cause distinctive epigenomic histone modification changes[39] and transcriptional reprogramming[38] thus induce distinct clinical phenotypes.

Traditional heteroplasmy detection using Sanger sequencing has limited sensitivity of about 20%. The NGS technology readily pushed the detection limit to 1% and, for ultradeep sequencing, pushing the power to detect low-level of heteroplasmy down to 0.01%,[40,41] so now NGS has replaced Sanger sequencing as the mainstream high throughput heteroplasmy detection strategy. There are multiple NGS-based heteroplasmy estimation analytical methods for online and standalone use. MToolBox can be run online at the MSeqDR website or as a standalone package. MToolBox, accepts different NGS data formats to provide a complete suite of analytical functions, including heteroplasmy estimation, haplogroup prediction, variant annotation, and prioritization. The MToolBox package works on both WGS and WES data. The mtDNA-Server[42] (https://mtdna-server.uibk.ac.at) supports web-based analysis of either single/paired-end FASTQ or BAM files in batch mode. The complete workflow includes BAM generation and heteroplasmy detection. The mtDNA-Server detects heteroplasmy to the 1% level with perfect specificity. Other tools include MitoSeek[43] and MitoSuite.[44] The number of heteroplasmic calls, number of congruent pairs between samples, and concordance between heteroplasmy calls using different tools vary, so further bioinformatics development and protocol evaluation are needed to standardize the heteroplasmy analysis performance and quality control metrics for clinical assay development and use. The super high sensitivity of NGS assays generally improves the diagnosis of mitochondrial diseases and the quality of genetic counseling, but may lead to difficulty in confirming very low heteroplasmy mtDNA variations and thus uncertainty in the diagnosis accuracy and consistency. For example, a tool was developed to produce corrected m.3243A>G heteroplasmy levels in muscle based on patient age and quantification in peripheral tissues of blood or uroepithelial cells[45] (https://newcastle-mito-apps.shinyapps.io/m3243ag_heteroplasmy_tool/).

HAPLOGROUP AND PHYLOGENY: IMPLICATIONS IN PATHOGENICITY INTERPRETATION

Haplotypes are sets of single nucleotide variants and/or small indels found within a genomic region of an individual when compared with the reference genome. Because of the lack of recombination among mitochondrial genomes, mtDNA haplotypes cluster together in the mtDNA phylogeny tree forming mtDNA haplogroups. The haplogroup-determining mtDNA variants are homoplasmic variants that are associated with particular maternal lineages that evolve as humans migrated across the globe. In addition to the importance of mitochondrial haplogroups for population genetics, they have also been shown to be associated with a number of rare and common diseases, such as Leber's hereditary optic neuropathy[46] and Parkinson disease.[47] The mtDNA haplogroup to which an individual's haplotype belongs must be considered when assessing a potentially pathogenic mtDNA variant. Accurate mitochondrial haplogroups determination is critical for population genetics and human disease diagnosis and research.

Several tools are available for automated mitochondrial haplogroup assignment. Phy-Mer[48] is a Python software package using a k-mer approach to do reference-free and alignment-free haplogroup classification. Phy-Mer supports input data in FASTA, FASTQ, or BAM formats, and supports variant calls as input data as well in either HGVS or VCF formats. It can be used online at the MSeqDR website MSeqDR (https://mseqdr.org/phymer.php), thus enabling analysis of mtDNA variants in conjunctions with nuclear variants via other tools developed and hosted by MSeqDR such as Quick-Mitome (https://mseqdr.org/qm.php). It performs equally well with the leading haplogroup classifier, HaploGrep,[49] while avoiding difficulties and errors in preparing the variant input in required formats and notations for running conventional variant-based tools like HaploGrep. MToolBox has comparable performance as Phy-Mer for haplogroup determination and is also available for online use at the MSeqDR website.

Other tools are reference based, requiring mitochondrial variants to be detected with a third-party aligner and a variant caller, and then the variants must be properly named according to certain notations before they can be compared with the haplogroup determining polymorphisms that are defined by PhyloTree[50] (http://www.phylotree.org/). Among them, HaploGrep[49] is currently the most popular one; other tools include MitoTool.[51]

For clinical interpretation, haplogroup markers are by definition benign. Unlike interpretation of nDNA variants, considering mtDNA phylogeny in conjugation with minor allele frequencies is critical for proper mtDNA variant interpretation. A particular mtDNA variant that may be a haplogroup marker or haplogroup-associated variant for 1 haplogroup may be associated with disease manifestations in the setting of other haplogroups.[52,53] For this reason, the MSeqDR-mvTool provides haplogroup 7information when annotating variants and allows browsing deeply annotated haplogroup-defining variants of all haplogroups with population frequency and in silico pathogenicity predictions with 1 click (https://mseqdr.org/mv4phylotree.php).[23]

SPECIFICATIONS OF THE AMERICAN COLLEGE OF MEDICAL GENETICS/ ASSOCIATION OF MOLECULAR PATHOLOGY STANDARDS AND GUIDELINES FOR MITOCHONDRIAL DNA VARIANT INTERPRETATION

As mentioned elsewhere in this article, pathogenicity interpretation of mtDNA variant has to give special considerations to unique features of the mtDNA genome, including variant heteroplasmy, threshold effect, absence of splicing, presence of haplogroups, and maternal inheritance. Currently, there is a lack of standards for mtDNA variant assessment, which leads to inconsistencies in clinical variant pathogenicity reporting. An international working group of mtDNA experts was assembled within the MSeqDR Consortium and sought Expert Panel status from ClinGen. This group reviewed the 2015 American College of Medical Genetic and Association of Molecular Pathology standards and guidelines[54] that are widely used for the clinical interpretation of nDNA sequence variants and provided further specifications for additional and specific guidance related to mtDNA variant classification. The 2015 American College of Medical Genetics/Association of Molecular Pathology variant interpretation guidelines were critically reviewed and specified for application in mtDNA variant assessment. These expert panel–based consensus specifications allow for consistent consideration of the unique aspects of the mtDNA genome that directly influence variant assessment, including addressing mtDNA genome composition and structure, haplogroups and phylogeny, maternal inheritance, heteroplasmy, and functional analyses unique to mtDNA, as well specifications for the use of mtDNA genomic databases and computational algorithms. It is expected that the guideline will be published and available soon.

MSeqDR FOR MITOCHONDRIAL DNA ANALYSIS AND MITOCHONDRIAL DISEASE DIAGNOSIS

MSeqDR is a comprehensive, continuously updated, and fully integrated genotype–phenotype data resource for the mitochondrial disease community, enabled by close collaborations among mitochondrial disease researchers and with several mitochondrial community resources, including MITOMAP and HmtDB.[22]

For genotype–disease association, the MSeqDR-LSDB is a continuously curated database of 280 mitochondrial diseases, more than 15,000 pathogenicity-assessed variants from 1500 genes related to mitochondrial functions, including more than 290 known disease genes curated by MSeqDR experts.

On the phenotypic side, the MSeqDR Disease Portal and Phenome backend are built on phenotype–disease–gene variant association data from Human Phenotype Ontology,[55] OMIM,[56] CTDBase,[57] Monarch Initiative and Mondo,[58] MedGen (https://www.ncbi.nlm.nih.gov/medgen/), ClinVar,[59] and DisGeNET.[60] The MSeqDR pseudo case registry has assembled more than 700 rare Leigh disease cases, 700 Leber's hereditary optic neuropathies and other mitochondrial disease cases mined from literature. The anonymous case-level data ere mapped from the usually free-text descriptions of clinical phenotypes into the most corresponding HPO phenotype ontology terms.

MSeqDR runs a full suite of bioinformatics tools to annotate, analyze, and interpret mtDNA and nuclear genome variants at whole genome and exome to single variant levels. For mtDNA data, the suite of online bioinformatics tools that are freely available consists of MSeqDR-mvTool, Phy-Mer, and MToolBox (HmtDB). They support mtDNA variant deep annotation and pathogenicity analysis (mvTool), haplogroup determination (Phy-Mer and MToolBox), and heteroplasmy calculation (MToolBox) with inputs in raw FASTQ, FASTA, and BAM formats. The mvTool annotates each mtDNA variant with the popular in silico predictions, including PolyPhen, SIFT, CADD score, and HmtDB's protein and RNA gene variant predictions. Additionally, mvTool provides pathogenicity classifications from MSeqDR, Mitomap, HmtDB, ClinVar, COSMIC, and ICGC (for somatic variants). The mvTool supports all 7 mtDNA variant nomenclatures and converts variants to standard rCRS- and HGVS-based nomenclatures. The web interface and 'mvTool API' support online and programmatic access using inputs in VCF, HGVS, or classical mtDNA variant nomenclatures. The results are reported as either hyperlinked HTML tables or downloadable files in JSON, Excel, and VCF formats. The estimated population allele frequencies are based on 40,000 additional germline mtDNA genomes, in addition to the 50,000 full-length mtDNA genomes compiled and curated by MitoMap and HmtDB.

For nDNA data, the Quick-Mitome variant interpretation platform is built on a proven phenotype-driven interpretation pipeline used in a clinical diagnostic setting at the Children's Hospital Los Angeles. It consisted of automatic online WES/WGS variant prioritization using Exomiser,[61] deep variant annotation with disease context, and variant data from MSeqDR, Mitomap, Hmtdb, Phylotree, ClinVar, dbNSFP,[62] VEP, and gnomAD population allele frequency.[63] The unified report summarizes the Exomiser ranking and cross-links all variants and genes to relevant MSeqDR, HPO and OMIM resources.

Clinical bioinformatics continues to evolve, following the technological advancements, so are the needs for improved bioinformatics tools for precise diagnosis of genetic diseases, including and represented by the family of highly heterogeneous family of mitochondrial diseases with genetic etiology of dual genome origin. As such, we anticipate the continuous emergence of new bioinformatics tools and methods, along with the continuous improvements of both nDNA and mtDNA specific references and databases. In doing so, it requires collective and cohesive efforts from disease domain experts and bioinformaticians across the globe, again as exemplified by the MSeqDR consortium.

DISCLOSURE

This work was supported by the United Mitochondrial Disease Foundation (UMDF) and the National Institutes of Health (U54-NS078059, U41-HG006834, and U24 HD093483-01).

REFERENCES

1. Gargis AS, Kalman L, Bick DP, et al. Good laboratory practice for clinical next-generation sequencing informatics pipelines. Nat Biotechnol 2015;33:689–93.
2. Wallace DC. Mitochondrial genetic medicine. Nat Genet 2018;50:1642–9.
3. Wallace DC, Chalkia D. Mitochondrial DNA genetics and the heteroplasmy conundrum in evolution and disease. Cold Spring Harb Perspect Biol 2013; 5(11):a021220.
4. McCormick EM, Zolkipli-Cunningham Z, Falk MJ. Mitochondrial disease genetics update: recent insights into the molecular diagnosis and expanding phenotype of primary mitochondrial disease. Curr Opin Pediatr 2018;30(6):714–24.
5. Wallace DC. Mitochondrial DNA variation in human radiation and disease. Cell 2015;163(1):33–8.
6. Stewart JB, Chinnery PF. The dynamics of mitochondrial DNA heteroplasmy: implications for human health and disease. Nat Rev Genet 2015;16(9):530–42.
7. McCormick E, Place E, Falk MJ. Molecular genetic testing for mitochondrial disease: from one generation to the next. Neurotherapeutics 2013;10(2):251–61.
8. Triska P, Kaneva K, Merkurjev D, et al. Landscape of germline and somatic mitochondrial DNA mutations in pediatric malignancies. Cancer Res 2019;79(7): 1318–30.
9. Calvo SE, Compton AG, Hershman SG, et al. Molecular diagnosis of infantile mitochondrial disease with targeted next-generation sequencing. Sci Transl Med 2012;4(118):118ra10.
10. Lieber DS, Calvo SE, Shanahan K, et al. Targeted exome sequencing of suspected mitochondrial disorders. Neurology 2013;80:1762–70.
11. Ohtake A, Murayama K, Mori M, et al. Diagnosis and molecular basis of mitochondrial respiratory chain disorders: exome sequencing for disease gene identification. Biochim Biophys Acta 2014;1840:1355–9.
12. Pronicka E, Piekutowska-Abramczuk D, Ciara E, et al. New perspective in diagnostics of mitochondrial disorders: two years' experience with whole-exome sequencing at a national paediatric centre. J Transl Med 2016;14:174.
13. Wortmann SB, Koolen DA, Smeitink JA, et al. Whole exome sequencing of suspected mitochondrial patients in clinical practice. J Inherit Metab Dis 2015;38: 437–43.

14. Haack TB, Danhauser K, Haberberger B, et al. Exome sequencing identifies ACAD9 mutations as a cause of complex I deficiency. Nat Genet 2010;42(12): 1131–4.

15. Neveling K, Feenstra I, Gilissen C, et al. A post-hoc comparison of the utility of Sanger sequencing and exome sequencing for the diagnosis of heterogeneous diseases. Hum Mutat 2013;34:1721–6.

16. Kremer L, Bader D, Mertes C, et al. Genetic diagnosis of Mendelian disorders via RNA sequencing. Nat Commun 2017;8:15824.

17. Cummings BB, Marshall JL, Tukiainen T, et al. Improving genetic diagnosis in Mendelian disease with transcriptome sequencing. Sci Transl Med 2017;9: eaal5209.

18. Clark MM, Hildreth A, Batalov S, et al. Diagnosis of genetic diseases in seriously ill children by rapid whole-genome sequencing and automated phenotyping and interpretation. Sci Transl Med 2019;11(489) [pii:eaat6177].

19. Ruiz-Pesini E, Lott MT, Procaccio V, et al. An enhanced MITOMAP with a global mtDNA mutational phylogeny. Nucleic Acids Res 2007;35:D823–8.

20. Clima R, Preste R, Calabrese C, et al. HmtDB 2016: data update, a better performing query system and human mitochondrial DNA haplogroup predictor. Nucleic Acids Res 2017;45:D698–706.

21. Preste R, Vitale O, Clima R, et al. HmtVar: a new resource for human mitochondrial variations and pathogenicity data. Nucleic Acids Res 2019;47(D1): D1202–10.

22. Shen L, Diroma MA, Gonzalez M, et al. MSeqDR: a centralized knowledge repository and bioinformatics web resource to facilitate genomic investigations in mitochondrial disease. Hum Mutat 2016;37(6):540–8.

23. Shen L, Attimonelli M, Bai R, et al. MSeqDR mvTool: a mitochondrial DNA Web and API resource for comprehensive variant annotation, universal nomenclature collation, and reference genome conversion. Hum Mutat 2018;39:806–10.

24. Ding J, Sidore C, Butler TJ, et al. Assessing mitochondrial DNA Variation and copy number in lymphocytes of ~2,000 Sardinians using tailored sequencing analysis tools. PLoS Genet 2015;11(7):e1005306.

25. Tadaka S, Katsuoka F, Ueki M, et al. 3.5KJPNv2: an allele frequency panel of 3552 Japanese individuals including the X chromosome. Hum Genome Var 2019;6:28.

26. Glusman G, Caballero J, Mauldin DE, et al. Kaviar: an accessible system for testing SNV novelty. Bioinformatics 2011;27(22):3216–7.

27. Ghosh R, Oak N, Plon SE. Evaluation of in silico algorithms for use with ACMG/AMP clinical variant interpretation guidelines. Genome Biol 2017;18:225.

28. Bris C, Goudenege D, Desquiret-Dumas V, et al. Bioinformatics tools and databases to assess the pathogenicity of mitochondrial DNA variants in the field of next generation. Front Genet 2018;9:632.

29. Castellana S, Rónai J, Mazza T. MitImpact: an exhaustive collection of precomputed pathogenicity predictions of human mitochondrial non-synonymous variants. Hum Mutat 2015;36(2):E2413–22.

30. Calabrese C, Simone D, Diroma MA, et al. MToolBox: a highly automated pipeline for heteroplasmy annotation and prioritization analysis of human mitochondrial variants in high-throughput sequencing. Bioinformatics 2014;30:3115–7.

31. Castellana S, Fusilli C, Mazzoccoli G, et al. High-confidence assessment of functional impact of human mitochondrial non-synonymous genome variations by APOGEE. PLoS Comput Biol 2017;13:e1005628.

32. Martin-Navarro A, Gaudioso-Simon A, Alvarez-Jarreta J, et al. Machine learning classifier for identification of damaging missense mutations exclusive to human mitochondrial DNA-encoded polypeptides. BMC Bioinformatics 2017;18:158.

33. Sonney S, Leipzig J, Lott MT, et al. Predicting the pathogenicity of novel variants in mitochondrial tRNA with MitoTIP. PLoS Comput Biol 2017;13:e1005867.

34. Niroula A, Vihinen M. PON-mt-tRNA: a multifactorial probability-based method for classification of mitochondrial tRNA variations. Nucleic Acids Res 2016;44:2020–7.

35. Elson JL, Smith PM, Greaves LC, et al. The presence of highly disruptive 16S rRNA mutations in clinical samples indicates a wider role for mutations of the mitochondrial ribosome in human disease. Mitochondrion 2015;25:17–27.

36. Smith PM, Elson JL, Greaves LC, et al. The role of the mitochondrial ribosome in human disease: searching for mutations in 12S mitochondrial rRNA with high disruptive potential. Hum Mol Genet 2014;23:949–67.

37. Gorman GS, Chinnery PF, DiMauro S, et al. Mitochondrial diseases. Nat Rev Dis Primers 2016;2:16080.

38. Picard M, Zhang J, Hancock S, et al. Progressive increase in mtDNA 3243A>G heteroplasmy causes abrupt transcriptional reprogramming. Proc Natl Acad Sci U S A 2014;111(38):E4033–42.

39. Kopinski PK, Janssen KA, Schaefer PM, et al. Regulation of nuclear epigenome by mitochondrial DNA heteroplasmy. Proc Natl Acad Sci U S A 2019;116:16028–35.

40. Schmitt MW, Kennedy SR, Salk JJ, et al. Detection of ultra-rare mutations by next-generation sequencing. Proc Natl Acad Sci U S A 2012;109:14508–13.

41. Ahn EH, Hirohata K, Kohrn BF, et al. Detection of ultra-rare mitochondrial mutations in breast stem cells by duplex sequencing. PLoS One 2015;10:e0136216.

42. Weissensteiner H, Forer L, Fuchsberger C, et al. mtDNA-Server: next-generation sequencing data analysis of human mitochondrial DNA in the cloud. Nucleic Acids Res 2016;44:W64–9.

43. Guo Y, Li C-I, Sheng Q, et al. Very low-level heteroplasmy mtDNA variations are inherited in humans. J Genet Genomics 2013;40:607–15.

44. Ishiya K, Ueda S. MitoSuite: a graphical tool for human mitochondrial genome profiling in massive parallel sequencing. PeerJ 2017;5:e3406.

45. Grady JP, Pickett SJ, Ng YS, et al. mtDNA heteroplasmy level and copy number indicate disease burden in m.3243A>G mitochondrial disease. EMBO Mol Med 2018;10:e8262.

46. Genasetti A, Valentino ML, Carelli V, et al. Assessing heteroplasmic load in Leber's hereditary optic neuropathy mutation 3460G->A/MT-ND1 with a real-time PCR quantitative approach. J Mol Diagn 2007;9:538–45.

47. Hudson G, Nalls M, Evans JR, et al. Two-stage association study and meta-analysis of mitochondrial DNA variants in Parkinson disease. Neurology 2013;80:2042–8.

48. Navarro-Gomez D, Leipzig J, Shen L, et al. Phy-Mer: a novel alignment-free and reference-independent mitochondrial haplogroup classifier. Bioinformatics 2015;31:1310–2.

49. Weissensteiner H, Pacher D, Kloss-Brandstatter A, et al. HaploGrep 2: mitochondrial haplogroup classification in the era of high-throughput sequencing. Nucleic Acids Res 2016;44:W58–63.

50. van Oven M, Kayser M. Updated comprehensive phylogenetic tree of global human mitochondrial DNA variation. Hum Mutat 2009;30:E386–94.

51. Fan L, Yao YG. MitoTool: a web server for the analysis and retrieval of human mitochondrial DNA sequence variations. Mitochondrion 2011;11:351–6.
52. Brown MD, Torroni A, Reckord CL, et al. Phylogenetic analysis of Leber's hereditary optic neuropathy mitochondrial DNA's indicates multiple independent occurrences of the common mutations. Hum Mutat 1995;6(4):311–25.
53. Wei W, Gomez-Duran A, Hudson G, et al. Background sequence characteristics influence the occurrence and severity of disease-causing mtDNA mutations. PLoS Genet 2017;13(12):e1007126.
54. Richards S, Aziz N, Bale S, et al. Standards and guidelines for the interpretation of sequence variants: a joint consensus recommendation of the American College of medical genetics and genomics and the association for molecular Pathology. Genet Med 2015;17:405–23.
55. Köhler S, Carmody L, Vasilevsky N, et al. Expansion of the human phenotype ontology (HPO) knowledge base and resources. Nucleic Acids Res 2019; 47(D1):D1018–27.
56. Hamosh A, Scott AF, Amberger JS, et al. Online mendelian inheritance in man (OMIM), a knowledgebase of human genes and genetic disorders. Nucleic Acids Res 2015;33(DI):D514–7.
57. Davis AP, Grondin CJ, Lennon-Hopkins K, et al. The comparative toxicogenomics database's 10th year anniversary: update 2015. Nucleic Acids Res 2015; 43(Database issue):D914–20.
58. Mungall CJ, McMurry JA, Köhler S, et al. The Monarch Initiative: an integrative data and analytic platform connecting phenotypes to genotypes across species. Nucleic Acids Res 2017;45:D712–22.
59. Landrum MJ, Lee JM, Riley GR, et al. ClinVar: public archive of relationships among sequence variation and human phenotype. Nucleic Acids Res 2014; 42(DI):D980–5.
60. Piñero J, Bravo À, Queralt-Rosinach N, et al. A comprehensive platform integrating information on human disease-associated genes and variants. Nucleic Acids Res 2017;45:D833–9.
61. Smedley D, Jacobsen JO, Jäger M, et al. Next-generation diagnostics and disease-gene discovery with the Exomiser. Nat Protoc 2015;10(12):2004–15.
62. Liu X, Wu C, Li C, et al. dbNSFP v3.0: a one-stop database of functional predictions and annotations for human non-synonymous and splice site SNVs. Hum Mutat 2016;37:235–41.
63. Karczewski KJ, Francioli LC, Grace T, et al. Variation across 141,456 human exomes and genomes reveals the spectrum of loss-of-function intolerance across human protein-coding genes. bioRxiv 531210. https://doi.org/10.1101/531210.

Bioinformatics in Clinical Genomic Sequencing

Matthew S. Lebo, PhD[a,b,c,]*, Limin Hao, PhD[a], Chiao-Feng Lin, PhD[a], Arti Singh, MS[a]

KEYWORDS

- Genome sequencing • Exome sequencing • Alignment • Variant calling • Annotation
- Filtration • Validation • Bioinformatic infrastructure

KEY POINTS

- Clinical bioinformatics encompasses generating raw sequence data from the machine through identifying reportable variants.
- Throughout the process, important quality control metrics are tracked based on the data, including the completeness of coverage across the region of interest for the assay.
- The process starts by taking raw sequence data, aligning it to a reference genome, and identifying variants based on the quality of the reads and the base pair calls.
- Variants are then annotated and filtered using a variety of features, including gene, transcript, Human Genome Variation Society nomenclature, population frequency, and presence in databases.
- In a clinical setting, a thorough validation of each of the components of the bioinformatics pipeline is critical, as is a detailed understanding of infrastructure, privacy, and security requirements.

INTRODUCTION

With the onset of high-throughput sequencing technologies, molecular genetic pathology has emerged from a visual-based specialty to an informatics-driven specialty. The increasing capabilities and reduced costs of sequencers, data computation, and data storage have enabled large-scaled sequencing (exomes and genomes) to be accessible to a wide range of patients. These include diagnosis of rare genetic conditions, in depth analysis of tumor–normal pairs, and screening of ostensibly healthy

This article originally appeared in *Advances in Molecular Pathology*, Volume 1, 2018.
Disclosure: The authors have nothing to disclose.
[a] Bioinformatics and Laboratory of Molecular Medicine, Partners Personalized Medicine, 65 Landsdowne Street, Cambridge, MA 02139, USA; [b] Pathology, Harvard Medical School, 25 Shattuck Street, Boston, MA 02115, USA; [c] Pathology, Brigham and Women's Hospital, 75 Francis Street, Boston, MA 02115, USA
* Corresponding author.
E-mail address: mlebo@bwh.harvard.edu

individuals. The increasing amount of data has also raised the profile of the burgeoning field of clinical bioinformatics. This article details the processes underlying clinical bioinformatics in the current molecular genetics workflow and provides the reader with a basic framework of the requirements needed to implement clinical bioinformatics in genomic sequencing.

SIGNIFICANCE

Although informatics is important in many aspects of laboratory testing, this article is focused on the computation, parsing, and analysis from sequencing machines through a final filtered set of variants. On the front end, the descriptions are most relevant for high-throughput genomic sequencing technologies (often referred to as next-generation sequencing [NGS]), although traditional sequencing machines have some commonalities. On the back end, this article stops short of the process of variant interpretation, although the software required for variant interpretation may depend on the clinical bioinformatics processes that come before it.

Overall Workflow

The typical clinical bioinformatics process can be seen in **Fig. 1**. The process can roughly be broken down into primary, secondary, and tertiary analysis. Primary analysis refers to the algorithms associated to the sequencing machines that convert the raw sequence reads to a string of As, Cs, Ts, and Gs. Secondary analysis details the mapping, or alignment, of these sequence reads onto the reference genomic sequence and then variant calling, or the identification of differences between the individual's sequence and the reference genome. Tertiary analysis involves the steps needed to properly interpret the sequence variants identified, and includes annotating and filtering the identified variants to find clinically relevant variation. Underlying all steps within the clinical bioinformatics process are the quality control metrics that determine the completeness, robustness, and reliability of the generated data.

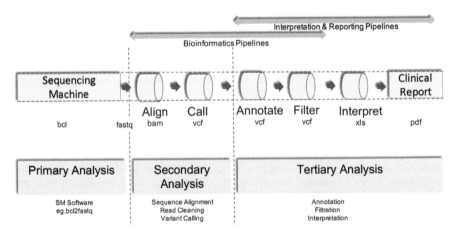

Fig. 1. Overview of bioinformatics processes in clinical genomic sequencing. This figure outlines the process for a data sample from the sequencing machine to clinical report. Detailed are the key steps in the process as well as some of the standard file types used in the pipeline.

Primary Analysis

Primary analysis algorithms are provided by the sequencing manufacturer to transform the raw data generated from the sequencing machine into interpretable sequence. Because the raw data are imperfect, the algorithms also contain associated quality metrics detailing the likelihood of each base call being correct. Different sequence manufacturers, techniques, and chemistries have different error patterns and error rates. Therefore, the error composition may not be identical from one sequence vendor to another. The sequence data are typically returned as fastq or ubam files (**Table 1**). These file types contain information on the sequence identified in each read, a per-base assignment of the quality of that variant, as well as data corresponding with the sequence read itself. Note that some techniques sequence 2 sides of a smaller sequencing fragment. This method, called paired-end

Table 1		
Common Data File Formats Used in Clinical Bioinformatics Tools		
File Type	**Link to Standard**	**Uses**
FASTA	https://fasta.bioch. virginia.edu/fasta_ www2/fasta_ intro.shtml	Originally the format of the input file for FASTA, which "Compares a protein sequence to another protein sequence or to a protein database, or a DNA sequence to another DNA sequence or a DNA library." It is most commonly used for storing reference genome sequences.
FASTQ	http://maq.sourceforge. net/fastq.shtml	It stores sequences and Phred qualities in a single file.
SAM (Sequence Alignment Map)	https://samtools. github.io/hts-specs/SAMv1.pdf	It is a tab-delimited text format consisting of a header section, which is optional, and an alignment section.
BAM/BAI	http://samtools. github.io/hts-specs/SAMv1.pdf	Binary form of SAM. BAI is BAM index file.
uBAM (unmapped BAM)	https://gatkforums. broadinstitute. org/gatk/ discussion/6484	Similar to BAM, because it maintains metadata, but with raw unmapped read sequences.
CRAM/CRAI	https://samtools. github.io/hts-specs/CRAMv3.pdf	CRAM is a more compressed version of aligned reads than BAM. Use of a CRAM file requires accessing the reference genome the reads were aligned to. CRAI is CRAM index file.
VCF/BCF	https://samtools. github.io/hts-specs/VCFv4.2.pdf	It contains metainformation lines, a header line, and then data lines each containing information about a position in the genome. The format also can contain genotype information on samples for each position. BCF is binary form of VCF.
BED (browser extensible data)	http://genome.ucsc. edu/FAQ/ FAQformat#format1	Originally designed for displaying annotation data on a genome browser. It became widely used for describing features over sequence intervals. Not to be confused with PLINK BED, which is binary ped for individual genotype data.

sequencing, can help with alignment and accuracy of the sequences. For the purposes of primary analysis, it is critical for these files to include information on the mate-pair to best use these additional data.

Secondary Analysis

Secondary analysis involves the taking the original sequencing data, processing it using a variety of statistical algorithms, and producing a set of sequence reads mapped to a genome and identifying difference between the individual and the reference. As mentioned, this stage depends on a reference genome. The reference genome is a standard set of sequence contigs for a species that define the current knowledge of the most likely consensus sequence, represented as a fasta file (see **Table 1**). It provides both a standard and a coordinate system to ensure the downstream components are referencing the same position. Typically, clinical laboratories currently use either hg19/GRCh37 or GRCh38 (**Box 1, Table 2**).

Once a defined reference sequence is selected, the secondary analysis pipeline typically involves the following components (**Table 3** provides examples of commonly used software):

- Alignment—The process of mapping the specific reads found in the sequencer to the reference genome. This step uses the quality metrics present in the sequence read as well as the uniqueness or redundancy of the genomic sequence to determine the quality of the alignment.
- Sequence read cleanup—Depending on the sequencer and/or downstream algorithms, the original mapped reads may be adjusted or removed. Typical

---

Box 1
Discussion of Genomic Reference Sequences

The human genome reference sequence is critical to the underlying clinical genomic bioinformatics process, because it provides both the template for alignment and a coordinate system for ensuring proper annotation and comparison of variants. There are 2 major genome builds currently in use today (GRCh37 [also referred to as hg19] and GRCh38). The GRC sequences are maintained by the Genome Reference Consortium (h referring to human), which releases both the reference genome build and patches to the build. Although the GRCh38 is a few years old, GRCh37 is still primarily used in clinical laboratories as the underlying annotation sources are being aligned against GRCh38 (see **Table 5**). There is also numerous software available that will liftover, or translate, between the 2 coordinate systems for resources that are only available on a single build.[34–36]

Many research laboratories and some clinical laboratories have migrated to using GRCh38. There are some advantages to doing this, including fixing of errors in the underlying genome build. Additionally, GRCh38 has a large increase in the number of alternative loci. These loci are large regions of the genome in which there are multiple common haplotypes. These alternative loci may help to increase the accuracy of alignment for individuals who have these haplotypes, although they can also cause further confusion downstream in terms of annotation and variant calling. However, alignment and variant calling software have been updated to deal with these alternative loci. It is up to the laboratory to determine which genome build they will use in their assays and a thorough understanding of the pros and cons for either build is important in making this decision.

Related to genome build is the underlying transcript coordinate system used (see **Table 2**). RefSeq and Ensembl are 2 of the major sources for transcripts, but take different approaches. RefSeq is independent of the genome build, but then contains differences where there might be discrepancies. Ensembl transcripts are mapped to the genome build, but then depend on the genome build being used. Choosing which transcript system is most applicable for your laboratory should also consider these differences.

Table 2
Community Resources in Clinical Bioinformatics

Type	Name	Link
Reference genome	GRCh37 (hg19)/ GRCh38	https://www.ncbi.nlm.nih.gov/grc
Transcript/Gene	Ensembl	http://ensembl.org/info/genome/ genebuild/genome_annotation.html
	RefSeq/Entrez	https://www.ncbi.nlm.nih.gov/refseq/
	LRG	http://www.lrg-sequence.org/
	CCDS	https://www.ncbi.nlm.nih.gov/projects/ CCDS/CcdsBrowse.cgi
	UCSC	https://genome.ucsc.edu/cgi-bin/hgTables
Official Gene Names and Symbols	HUGO	https://www.genenames.org
Variant Nomenclature	HGVS	http://varnomen.hgvs.org/

examples include removing duplicate reads that may be sequencing artifacts or using a more specialized local alignment within some of the reads.

- Variant calling—Using the mapped reads, algorithms look for differences between these reads and the reference genome. These differences may be single nucleotides, or large structural variants, depending on the sequencing methodology. The quality of these variant calls is determined using the quality and abundance of the sequence reads.

Alignment

During the alignment phase, the sequence reads are mapped to the reference genome. These alignment algorithms use data from the quality of the specific base calls as well as specific parameters allowing for both mismatches and gaps as compared with the reference. In this regard, a longer sequence read tends to map more accurately, because it enables less ambiguity in the alignment as well being able to handle more individual-specific variation against the reference genome. Furthermore, mapping from paired-end sequences can use 1 read with a high likelihood of aligning to a particular region to anchor the other read that may have similarity with multiple regions of the genome. Alignment software also gives a statistical likelihood that the read maps to the genomic region predicted, and is often represented as mapping quality (**Table 4** provides definitions of quality metrics). Mapping quality represents the uniqueness of the region in the reference genome to which the read aligns, with regions not being able to uniquely map given a lower mapping quality score. See **Box 2** for a discussion of difficult genomic regions.

Sequence read cleanup

There are often additional tools used after the alignment step to further process and clean the reads that have been mapped. Examples include the following.

- Aligned reads will get sorted by genomic position to enable faster processing in the downstream steps.
- For some methods, reads that are exact copies are likely to be duplicates of the original raw data and could skew variant calling if more than 1 read is included.
- Many algorithms realign certain regions, including around suspected indels, where the default settings in the alignment step may not be reliable.

Table 3
Examples of Popular Software Used in Secondary Analysis

Software Class	Name	Use	Ref
Alignment	BWA-SW	Alignment for shorter reads	Li & Durbin [42], 2009
	BWA-MEM	Alignment for longer reads (>100 bp)	Li & Durbin [43], 2010
	Novoalign	Commercial alignment software	[44]
Manipulating mapped sequence read files	Picard Tools [45], Samtools [46], and GATK [47]	were all developed very early when next-generation sequencing was not so pervasive. They have been kept up to date with the advancement of sequencing technology and data processing best practices. They overlap on functions for frequently used manipulation. Samtools was implemented in C and Picard and GATK in Java.	
Manipulating and analyzing VCF files	Both BCFtools [48] and VCFtools [49] accept BCF and VCF files. The two have a highly overlapping set of functions yet each has its distinctive analytical features.		
SNV and indel calling	BCFtools/Samtools	Its variant calling is not used as widely as its other versatile features.	Li [45], 2011
	GATK—UnifiedGenotyper	Earlier version of GATK variant caller. Gradually gives way to HaplotypeCaller.	McKenna et al, [46] 2010
	GATK—HaplotypeCaller	Its local de novo assembly made the local realignment step that was required for UnifiedGenotyper redundant and intrinsically phases genotype calls to some extent.	Poplin et al, [47] 2017
	Freebayes	Bayesian haplotype-based. Its ability to use prior information and nonuniform genome-wide ploidy provided by users makes it more effective in analyzing genomes having particular properties.	Garrison & Marth [48], 2012
SV and CNV calling	Pindel	Detects large deletions and medium insertions by finding breakpoints in the unmapped pair-end read.	Ye et al, [49] 2009
	BreakDancer	One of very early SV callers. Detects SV by analyzing anomalous mapped read pairs.	Fan et al, [50] 2014
	GenomeStrip	Requires ≥20 samples. Analyzes a combination of read depth, read length, and read mate-pairing.	Handsaker et al, [51] 2015
	Manta	Illumina's SV and medium indels caller for germline and somatic analysis.	Chen et al, [52] 2016
	XHMM	CNV calling for exome data.	Fromer & Purcell [53], 2014
	VisCap	CNV calling for panel data.	Pugh et al, [54] 2016

Manipulating genomic intervals	bedtools	Touted as a Swiss Army Knife of tools for genome arithmetical, it is particularly useful for manipulating multiple bed (or other genomic interval format) files.	Quinlan [55], 2014
Variant call comparison	vcfeval	Can compare 2 different variant call files. Useful for validation.	Cleary et al, [56] 2015
Obtaining quality control metrics	FastQC	Provides metrics useful for assessing sequencing quality. Supports multiple platforms.	[57]
	verifybamID	Detects sample contaminations and swaps.	Jun et al, [58] 2012
	Picard Tools	Provides quality control metrics for various stages of secondary analysis.	[59]

Abbreviations: CNV, copy number variant; SNV, structural variant.

Table 4
Examples of Quality Metrics in Secondary Analysis

Name	Abbreviation	Definition
Read depth	DP	Depth of sequencing coverage at that position
Mapping quality	MQ	Mapping quality of specific position
Strand bias	SB	Measure of strand bias at that position
Variant call quality by depth	QD	Variant call quality normalized by depth
Quality score	QUAL	Confidence of any call at that position
Genotype call quality	GQ	Confidence in the genotyping call in an individual
Allele depth	AD	Coverage of specific variants at genomic position

- Some algorithms will adjust quality metrics using a set of variant calls most likely to be real.

Variant calling

Variant calling is perhaps both the most critical step in the clinical bioinformatics process as well as the biggest black box and most reliant on statistical modeling. The goal of variant calling is to identify all the instances where the individual's sequence is different as compared with the reference genome. These differences may be small (eg, single nucleotide variants [SNVs]) or may be very large (eg, multiple megabase deletions). Variant calling algorithms are often targeted to a class of variant (see examples elsewhere in this article and in **Table 3**), and even to a specific type of sequencing assay (eg, genome vs exome copy number variant calling). Detailed herein are some of the common variant types and approaches seen in genomic sequencing.

Box 2
Challenging Genomic Regions in Clinical Sequencing

There are certain regions of the genome that are complex and challenging to interrogate with the current sequencing modalities. These regions can cause decreases in accuracy during sequencing and are important to understand upfront in the assay development process. Difficult genomic regions are normally described as the following categories.

- Low complexity DNA regions can be simple repeats (microsatellites where a unit of 2 or 3 nucleotides repeat many times), poly-purine (strings of guanine or cytosine)/poly-pyrimidine (adenine or thymine) stretches, or regions of extremely high AT or GC content.

- Segmental duplication are large-scale chromosomal duplications. They can be remnants of whole genome duplication. Such regions have high similarity (homology).

- Low mappability. Mappability describes how sequence reads can be uniquely mapped/aligned to a region. This factor can vary depending on read lengths. The longer the reads are, the greater the overall mappability of a genome is.

- High or low guanine-cytosine (GC) content.

These categories can be somewhat related. For instance, both low-complexity regions and segmental duplications can lead to low mappability. Genomic regions with particularly high GC content are difficult to sequence owing to the stronger base pairing between G (guanine) and C (cytosine) than that of A (adenine) and T (thymine). This can lead to insufficient coverage. The Genome in a Bottle Consortium and the Global Alliance for Genomics and Health have defined a set of these regions that can be useful during benchmarking and validation of pipelines [37] and a similar resource has identified stretches of homology in clinically relevant genes that could cause issues in sequencing.[38]

Single nucleotide variants and small insertion/deletions SNVs and small insertion and/or deletion events (indels) are the smallest type of change identified in genomic sequencing assays. In this process, differences against the reference sequence are identified in the individual sequence reads. The quality metrics of the individual reads are combined for each of the reads overlapping that position to generate confidence in the call. In germline sequencing, heterozygous calls should have roughly one-half the reads with the variant call and homozygous calls should have all reads with the variant call. Owing to random stochastic processes, especially at low coverage depth, low-quality sequence reads, ambiguities in mapping, and challenges with indel detection, the actual fraction of reads with a variant call may be different.

In general, variant calling for SNVs is highly accurate (>99.5% sensitivity and specificity).[1] Indels, however, can prove more difficult. The longer the insertion/deletion event, the more challenging it is to map the read accurately. Additionally, if the indel even gets called at the end of the read, it is difficult for the aligner to know if this is a true variant or due to the reduced accuracy, in general, of nucleotide calls at the ends of reads. Other reasons may lead to more difficulty in calling SNVs/indels include the following.

- The variant lies in a challenging genomic region. For instance, regions with high homology are difficult to accurately map reads against. See **Box 2** for more details.
- The variant is near or part of a homopolymer stretch. This positioning can cause issues with alignment and changes in the homopolymer stretches may appear as SNVs.
- Complex insertion deletion events can often look to the aligner like separate variants.

Copy number variants and structural variants Genomic sequencing can also detect copy number variation (gains or losses of genomic sequence) and other types of structural variation (translocations, copy neutral insertions, inversions, fusions, chromothripsis, etc). These events can range from single exon copy number changes to megabase-sized events. However, the ability and methodologies used to detect these events depends entirely on the type of sequencing assay, the method for capturing genomic sequence, and other upstream sequencing assays.[2] For instance, exome and panel sequencing assays typically use one type of data (read depth) for calling copy number variants because breakpoints typically lie in intronic or intergenic sequences and they cannot use other methods that make use of breakpoint data. Similarly, exome- and panel-based assays do not detect other balanced structural variations, unless the assay is designed specifically to detect them (ie, fusion events in cancer or known, recurrent deletions), whereas genome sequencing can make use of both breakpoint and paired-end analysis to find these events.

Regions of homozygosity Depending on the size of the sequencing panel, one may be able to identify large stretches of the genome where the individual seems to only have homozygous variation (also referred to absence of heterozygosity or loss of heterozygosity). Although this may occur sporadically owing to the presence of only common variation in that region, larger stretches may in fact reflect disease-causing variation, for instance, uniparental disomy or an underlying rare homozygous pathogenic variant. Additionally, summing up these homozygosity stretches can indicate both degrees of consanguinity (in germline sequencing) and tumor progression (in somatic sequencing).

Genotyping from sequencing The benefit of high-throughput sequencing lies in the ability to scan large genomic regions for variation, including novel variation, and not being limited to previously discovered variation. However, there are times when it is critical to know not only if the individual has the variant, but also exactly what their genotype is at a specific position. Common examples here include pharmacogenomic variation and instances where the disease-associated variant is the reference allele (often seen in risk alleles, eg, the factor V Leiden allele in GRCh37). A standard vcf file will just contain variation against the reference, so the downstream processes may not be able to determine whether the absence of a call is due to lack of data or if the individual is truly homozygous reference. Therefore, genotyping these specific positions off the sequencing data can provide further confidence into the individual's exact genotype.

Tertiary Analysis

During tertiary analysis, the identified sequence variants are placed more broadly into the genomic and clinical context. Whereas secondary analysis ends with the identification of a genomic change (ie, a difference against the genomic reference), tertiary analysis enables the downstream systems and users to appropriately interpret the exact difference. This factor makes the process both difficult and critically important to make robust and complete, and provides its own challenges in validation (discussed elsewhere in this article).

Tertiary analysis can involve the following components.

- Annotation—The process of adding details to the identified genomic change, including gene, transcript, and nomenclature information. This gives the specific context and available knowledge for the variant of interest.
- Filtration/prioritization—In genomic sequencing, depending on what was targeted, one can identify hundreds, thousands, or even millions of variants. Filtration involves the process of using bioinformatic approaches and annotations to limit the number of variants that require manual review.
- Interpretation—Although the actual process of variant interpretation falls outside of the purview of clinical bioinformatics, the data and systems used for interpretation are entirely within scope. Thus, it is critical for this component to follow standard bioinformatic practices.

Annotation

After variant calling, the variants need to be annotated to assess their effects in biology, physiology, and clinical relevance. This analysis involves extracting available knowledge at the gene, transcript, protein, and regulatory levels from biological databases, as well as a detailed knowledge of the variant at the population and evolution levels to predict the effects and function of a variant. Prior clinical data and published literature are also mined to identify previous genetic information that may indicate disease association.

Gene/transcript annotation and Human Genome Variation Society nomenclature Clinical genomic interpretation today remains focused on coding content. Thus, at its basis, a variant is annotated with regard to the genes and transcripts in which it lies. These annotations place the variant in the context of the coding portion of the gene, and include variant effect (silent, nonsense, missense, frameshift, etc), variant location (exon, intron, untranslated region), and variant nomenclature. A gene can be expressed in multiple forms (transcripts) by alternative splicing. The position of a variant in a gene could affect all or only some of the transcripts. Different laboratories use different resources for determining transcripts (see **Table 2**) and different policies for determining the major transcript (ie, longest, most highly expressed, historic, or transcript with most clinically relevant variants).

Regarding variant nomenclature, the Human Genome Variation Society has developed and iterated on a sequence variant nomenclature system and its recommendations have been widely accepted as the standard, which provides a consistent and unambiguous description of sequence variants.[3] The representation of variants by these recommendations is described at the most basic DNA level and in relation to an accepted reference sequence. The type of reference sequences used is indicated by 6 letter prefixes—g, c, m, n, r, and p—corresponding with genomic DND, cDNA, mitochondrial DNA, noncoding RNA, RNA, and protein sequences. The more detailed recommendations can be seen at http://varnomen.hgvs.org/.

Population frequency Minor allele frequency is ratio of the count of a nonreference allele to total number of alleles of the same locus in a population. A low allele frequency implies rarity of the variant, which is usually thought as linked to disease, although this is not always the case. The aggregation of genome sequencing data (eg, 1000 Genome Project, Exome Aggregation Consortium, and Genome Aggregation Database) [4–6] allows the integration of hundreds of thousands of individuals to compute variant frequencies across different ethnicities. So far, variant frequencies have been computed in more than 20 races that are further clustered into subpopulations, such as Black, American, Ashkenazi Jewish, East Asian, non-Finnish European, Finnish, and South Asian. Laboratories will use the maximum of these minor allele frequencies across the subpopulations as an aid in filtration, with the assumption that a particular population does not have an increased incidence of a certain disease that would cause a higher subpopulation frequency.

The sequencing depth, also known as coverage, is an important indicator to evaluate the sequencing quality. It determines if absence of a variant is real or due to poor coverage at genomic location. Although the aggregated data provided precise allele frequency among human races, an average coverage data will facilitate assessing the quality of variant frequency.

Variant databases To annotate variants accurately and precisely, high-quality and reliable data sources are essential. These data sources can be public or commercially available. A list of datasets and databases is included in **Table 5**, which are selected by laboratories based on their availability, quality, and reliability. These resources often contain information on variant classification, disease association, relevant literature, and case history. They are crucial to determining the previous genetic information known about a variant.

Computational prediction algorithms and conservation There are many algorithms available that attempt to computationally predict the effect that a variant may have on a protein (ie, MutationAssessor, MutationTaster, PolyPhen2, REVEL [7–10]). Initial methods aimed to determine the potential impact of missense variation on a protein, whereas more recent, sophisticated algorithms attempt to predict the effect of any genomic change. In general, these algorithms predict benign variation better than pathogenic variation and still suffer from a high number of false calls. These tools often make use of conservation of the nucleotide or amino acid across species, where high conservation can be reflective of positive selection and thus likely functional consequence.

To implement variant annotation, a few software tools (ANNOVAR, SnpEff, VEP, Oncotator), among a long list of bioinformatics genome annotation tools, are commonly used (**Table 6**).[11–14] A more integrated annotation tool named WGSA

Table 5
Datasets and Databases for Variant Annotation

Dataset/ Database	Description	Features	GRCh37	GRCh38
dbSNP	A central repository for both SNP/indel polymorphisms.	Variant ID, location.	Yes	Yes
Human Gene Mutation Database (HGMD)	Repository for all known (published) gene lesions responsible for human inherited disease.	It provides gene symbol, cDNA sequence, genomic coordinates, HGVS nomenclature, missense/nonsense, splicing, regulatory, deletions/insertions, complex rearrangements, repeat variations.	Yes	Yes
ClinVar	Repository of human variants related to phenotypes with supporting evidence.	It provides identifiers, attributes of phenotype, description of the genotype/phenotype relationship, submission information, represented evidence, integrated data from multiple sources.	Yes	Yes
LOVD	Repository of gene-centered DNA variations, as well as storage of patient-centered data and NGS data.	It provides gene symbol, genomic position of variants, variants on genes, variants on transcripts, variants in a patient, all diseases associated with a gene, all screenings for a gene.	NA	NA
1000 Genome	A project to find genetic variants with frequencies of ≥1%.	Population frequency.	Yes	Yes
gnomAD	A resource aggregating both exome and genome sequencing data from a wide variety of large-scale sequencing projects.	Population frequency, coverage.	Yes	No
ExAC	Same as gnomAD.	Population frequency, coverage.	Yes	No
Alamut	A database that integrates NCBI, EBI, UCSC, HGVS nomenclature.	It provides annotations such as variant effect, splicing prediction, protein domain, functional prediction.	Yes	Yes
dbNSFP	A lightweight database of human nonsynonymous SNPs and their functional predictions.	It compiles prediction scores from SIFT, Polyphen2, LRT, MutationTaster, PhyloP and other related information for every potential nonsynonymous variant in the human genome. It also provides annotations of conservation values, function prediction.	Yes	Yes

Abbreviations: HGVS, Human Genome Variation Society; NGS, next-generation sequencing; SNP, single nucleotide polymorphism.

Table 6
Commonly Used Software of Variant Annotation

Software	Description	Functionality	Ref
ANNOVAR	An efficient software tool to use update-to-date information to functionally annotate genetic variants.	Gene-based, region-based, filter-based annotation.	Wang et al,[11] 2010
SnpEff	A variant annotation and effect prediction tool.	It annotates and predicts the effects of variants on genes.	Cingolani et al,[13] 2012
VEP	A variant effect predictor.	VEP determines the effect of variants on genes, transcripts and protein sequence, as well as regulatory regions.	McLaren et al,[12] 2016
Oncotator	A web application for annotating human genomic point mutations and indels with data relevant to cancer researchers.	Annotations are aggregated from Genomic Annotations, protein annotations, cancer variants annotations, and noncancer variant annotations.	Ramos et al,[14] 2015
WGSA	WGSA is an annotation pipeline for human genome resequencing studies, to facilitate the functional annotation step of whole genome sequencing.	It integrates the outputs from ANNOVAR, SnpEff, and VEP for gene-model based annotation. It also integrates multiple prediction scores, conservation scores, allele frequencies and disease related database for SNV-centric resources, as well as integrates multiple epigenomics projects for regulatory region-centric resources.	Liu et al,[15] 2016
CADD	CADD is a tool for scoring the deleteriousness of SNP/ indels variants in the human genome.	It integrates multiple annotations into one metric by contrasting variants that survived natural selection with simulated mutations. It is an algorithm designed to annotate both coding and noncoding variants.	Kircher et al,[60] 2014
DANN	A deep learning approach for annotating the pathogenicity of genetic variants.	Same as CADD.	Quang et al,[61] 2014

Abbreviations: CADD, combined annotation-dependent depletion; SNP, Single nucleotide polymorphism; SNV, single nucleotide variant; WGSA, WGS Annotator.

was relatively recently developed which integrates the outputs of other annotation approaches and combines other prediction scores, conservations scores, and knowledge of regulator region-centric resources to annotate variants.[15] The procedure of variant annotation for a sample is shown in **Fig. 2**.

Gene-level annotations The clinical effect of a variant is principally through affecting expression and function of the gene. If a protein plays a known function in human physiology, loss or alteration of the protein's function could lead to phenotypic consequences. It is, therefore, important to determine the likelihood that altering a protein will affect biological function. This analysis can be done by evaluating the evidence of a gene–disease association. The Clinical Genome Reference (ClinGen) has produced a framework and a team of curators for this task.[16] Additionally, it is important to know whether a gene can tolerate variation, particularly whether it can tolerate a loss-of-function variation, to know the likelihood of a specific variant having an impact. Computational resources examining how constrained a gene is against variation, including loss-of-function variation, have been developed and are widely used.[4,17,18]

Filtration/prioritization
After annotating the identified variants, one is left with thousands, tens of thousands, or even millions of variants to sort through. This scenario is obviously too challenging to perform manually and thus the bioinformatics processes must make use of the structured annotation data generated. The goal of the filtration component is to get to the minimal set of variants required to interpret for the assay (**Fig. 3**). In panel-based sequencing, this may be every variant identified in the regions or genes of interest, whereas in exome or genome sequencing this may be the smaller set of variants most likely to have clinical relevance.

The simplest filter mechanism, and the one used in nearly every assay, is to limit the variants to exons, genes, and/or regions of interest. These regions may be predefined by the assay or defined on the fly based on the individual's presentation. Either way, the goal is to limit the reviewed variants to those most likely to correspond with the indication for testing. A similar approach is to limit variants in exome and genome sequencing to the medical exome, or the set of approximately 2000 to 4500 genes with evidence of having a disease association.

Other common types of filtration approaches include the following. Often, multiple filters or combinations of filters are applied in each case. A more in-depth discussion on the tools used in tertiary analysis can be found in **Box 3** and some challenges can be found in **Box 4**.

- Genetics-based filtration—This includes sequencing a trio (proband and parents) and looking for compound heterozygous or homozygous variants in recessive conditions, or de novo variation in sporadic cases; sequencing multiple affected individuals to find variants in common; and sequencing a tumor/normal pair to identify somatically derived variation.

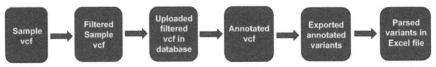

Fig. 2. Key steps of variant annotation. A sample vcf file is filtered through a bed file with regions of interest. The filtered vcf file is then uploaded into database and annotated. The annotated variants can then be managed in the software, or can be exported and examined externally, such as in Excel.

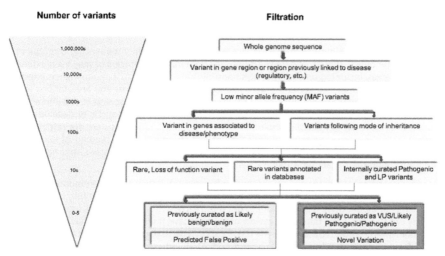

Fig. 3. Genomic sequencing filtration process. Example of a filtration workflow for identifying disease-associated variants from genomic sequencing. As more filters are applied, the smaller the number of variants that are kept for review. After variants are filtered in, they may have different classifications based on previous interpretation or quality metrics. Variants in green should be reviewed quickly, but can be discarded quickly. Variants in red will need a more thorough review process to determine if they meet reporting criteria. LP, likely pathogenic; VUS, variant of uncertain significance.

- Phenotype-based filtration—As mentioned, limiting the variant calls to those previously associated with the disease or present in genes with established disease causation. The gene-based approach captures all potential variation in the gene, whereas the variant-based approach relies on previously published information present in curated variant databases (eg, ClinVar [19]).

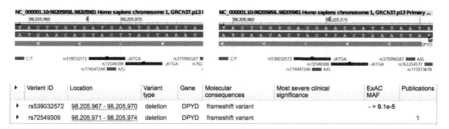

	Variant ID	Location	Variant type	Gene	Molecular consequences	Most severe clinical significance	ExAC MAF	Publications
▶	rs539032572	98,205,967 - 98,205,970	deletion	DPYD	frameshift variant		- = 9.1e-5	
▶	rs72549309	98,205,971 - 98,205,974	deletion	DPYD	frameshift variant			1

Fig. 4. A variant cannot be unambiguously placed at 1 specific location. A deletion of 1 unit (ATGA) of tandem repeats can be placed at 2 locations, which are represented by 2 database of single nucleotide polymorphisms (dbSNP) entries: (1) rs539032572: NC_00 0001.10:g.98205967_98205970delATGA and (2) rs72549309: NC_000001.10:g.98205 971_98205974delATGA. Both result in a frameshift. Deletion of either unit would be annotated as rs539032572 (*left align*) in vcf, whereas rs72549309 (*right align*) per Human Genome Variation Society (HGVS) guidelines. rs72549309 is cited in 1 publication on pharmacogenes. A researcher looking for its allele frequency in ExAC would not find any frequency information because the same ATGA deletion is represented by rs539032572 in ExAC, whose variants are natively stored in vcf. (*Adapted from* National Center for Biotechnology Information. Variation viewer. Available at: https://www.ncbi.nlm.nih.gov/variation/view/. Accessed April 17, 2018.)

Box 3
Resources for Tertiary Analysis

There are numerous bioinformatic software solutions for the tertiary sequencing component of clinical genomics. These software solutions may do part of the process or may even extend into other areas, including secondary analysis and clinical reporting. At a minimum, it is important for these solutions to contain a genomic database that can store the annotations in a robust way and that efficient searching or filtering can be performed against it. It is important to remember that, whether these systems are vendor supplied, open source, or developed in house, the molecular geneticist/pathologist and the clinical bioinformaticians are responsible for ensuring their accuracy. It is also critical to have a thorough understanding of how they work, including which data they are using, how that data have been parsed, and how they are performing their exact filtrations.

Another important aspect to consider for these softwares is that they offer a continuous learning environment. Typically, variants that are either parsed during a triage process or fully interpreted are seen on multiple cases. It is important to get these variant classifications back into the system so they can be used in the filtering or review of the next case. It is also useful to have the date of the initial interpretation to make sure the classification is up to date with the most recent knowledge. Similarly, it is useful to maintain a repository of all individuals who have been identified with a variant. This way, when a variant classification changes, it can be properly reflected in each of the previous cases and communicated to the clinicians if necessary.

- Variant-based filtration—This filtration strategy may be unbiased. It relies on using structured annotations to extract variants with certain features, including:
  - Rarity (low frequency or absence) in population databases;
  - Type of variation (ie, nonsense, missense mutations);

Box 4
Challenges in Annotation and Variant Nomenclature

Although annotation of variants in genomic sequencing is critical, there are often difficulties of which the molecular geneticist/pathologist needs to be aware. One of the most challenging aspects that can cause issues in annotation involved variant nomenclature and how variants are represented in different standards. For instance, although the Human Genome Variation Society provides rules for variant nomenclature, some of the rules are ambiguous, allow for multiple options, or have changed over time. Similarly, HUGO, the resource responsible for determining gene names and symbols, is often updating these symbols in real time, causing gene nomenclature to become inaccurate and obsolete. This factor makes accurately mapping the change identified in an individual to a change previously reported difficult at times.

One way to solve this issue is to ensure that all annotations involve the same standard. For instance, a common approach is to use vcf files to add annotations, because this approach can normalize the information to a single genomic change. However, this also can cause challenges. Namely, the vcf standard for indels is different than the Human Genome Variation Society standard for indels. Often, an indel occurs at a region where there is similar sequence context, because the variant cannot be unambiguously placed at one specific location (**Fig. 4**). In this case, the vcf standard is to shift the indel to the 5′ most position on the genomic reference (left align). The Human Genome Variation Society standard, however, has the indel shifted to the 3′ most position on the transcript (right align). Therefore, when the transcript is on the top (or positive) strand, the indels will be represented by different genomic positions. The Human Genome Variation Society standard also may use duplication or repeat nomenclature, which is not part of the vcf standard. Furthermore, the vcf standard does not allow for blank values for either the reference (ref) or variant (alternative; alt) fields, causing insertion and deletion events to be shifted by another position to account for the upstream nucleotide that is not part of the event. Accounting for these issues in the bioinformatics pipeline are possible, so it is important that the molecular geneticist/pathologist knows how they were implemented.

- Location of variant (ie, near splice site); and
- In silico predicted effects on function, structure, or evolutionary conservation.

Interpretation

The final stage in the clinical genomics workflow before reporting is providing a full interpretation of the identified variants, which entails using all available evidence to determine a variant's association with disease. Recent guidelines have detailed approaches for classifying both germline and somatic variation.[20,21] Although the actual interpretation falls outside of the purview of clinical bioinformatics, the software and resources used are often heavily driven by the informatics infrastructure, especially reliable and complete annotation of the data.[22] Therefore, an understanding of the interpretation workflow is critical to clinical bioinformatics. The number of possible annotations is often too numerous to completely consume manually and the bioinformatics workflow is responsible for paring those down into clinically meaningful subsets.

In the genomic workflow, there are often multiple different approaches to interpretation. As mentioned, the number of variants that come out of the pipeline cannot be all reviewed manually for each case. Therefore, filtration and other methods are needed to be able to parse through these variants while maintaining a high clinical rigor. This process includes the following.

- Preclassifying variation before identifying it in the laboratory. One use case would be relatively common pathogenic variation that one is likely to encounter during testing. Another use case would be variants that have high population frequency and no evidence for pathogenicity that can be classified as benign or likely benign.
- Triaging variants that come out of the filtration process. Even though the filtration process is geared toward extracting variants that are most likely to have clinical relevance, often variants get pulled in whose evidence is limited. These variants can be parsed through more quickly, assuming they do not meet requirements to be included on the clinical report.
- Full assessment of variant pathogenicity. For variants that may have clinical relevance, it is important to use a tool that pulls in all potentially relevant data and enables the molecular geneticist/pathologist to perform a thorough review and approve the final variant classification.

Quality Control Measures

The clinical bioinformatics process for genomic sequencing focuses on identifying and interpreting variation, but includes numerous additional components. Chief among these are analyzing the data at various steps for quality control measures, including what was done during the upstream laboratory process. The quality control metrics can help to determine the accuracy and completeness of the sequencing assay. Some common metrics can be found in **Table 7**. More specific use cases during the quality control process are detailed herein.

Coverage

In a NGS assay, coverage (often represented by depth) is a measure of the number of reads overlapping a position. Although the overall raw coverage of a base can be useful, most clinical metrics view coverage in terms of usable data or data that would be used to make a variant call. In this regard, coverage is often reduced to those reads where both the mapping quality of the entire read is high and the base quality for the specific position within that read is high. Coverage also often gets defined by 2 metrics:

Table 7		
Common Quality Control Metrics		
Type	**Metric**	**Definition**
Coverage	Average coverage	Average depth across all bases within ROI
	% completeness	% of bases within ROI at a minimum depth of coverage (ie, 15)
	% low covered regions	% of regions not meeting target coverage level
Sample identity	Contamination	Estimate of the number of reads that come from another individual or another species, such as bacteria
	% identity	Uniqueness of sample as compared with an orthogonal genotyping assay
Sequencing metrics	Total number of reads	Total number of raw read associated to the sample
	% reads passing filters	% of raw reads that pass filter metrics for being of sufficient quality
	% reads mapped	% of raw reads that map to reference genome
	% reads on target	% of raw reads that map to capture region (not used in genome sequencing)
	Insert size	In paired-end sequencing, the average distance between the 2 ends of the sequence
Variant metrics	Total number of variants	Total number of variants identified in ROI; should reflect control samples in ROI
	Ti/Tv ratio	Ratio of transitions to transversions. Should reflect control samples in ROI
	SNV/Indel ratio	Ratio of SNV to indel calls. Should reflect control samples in ROI
	Het/Hom ratio	Ratio of heterozygous variants to homozygous variants. Should reflect control samples in ROI

Abbreviations: ROI, region of interest; SNV, single nucleotide variant.

- Average coverage—Across all positions within the region of interest, the average number of usable reads that align; and
- Percent completeness—For a given coverage depth (ie, 15×), the percent of bases within the region of interest that have at least that coverage

These metrics can be measured at an exon, gene, panel, exome, or genome level. Typically, completeness is more informative owing to differences in sequencing ability because it more accurately reflects the overall ability to call variants.

Contamination
Owing to the generally high depth within clinical sequencing assays and the size of the sequencing assays, it is also possible to detect low level contamination in samples. This contamination may be due to other clinical samples in the laboratory, or my even be due to bacteria and other organisms. Depending on the specific assay and library preparation methods, it may be important to monitor sequencing runs for contamination, because a small amount may compromise variant calling.

Identity checking
Similarly, it is also important to ensure that the data from the sequencer and against which variant calling is occurring is correctly associated with the right individual. In this regard, it is possible to use both the sheer number of variants called and rare variation. Using the population frequency of potential variants, one can determine the uniqueness of a sample. Combining this information with a previous a separately run dataset (often a genotyping array or small sequencing assay), one can determine

that the data they are reviewing is from the individual from which it is suspected to have come.

Validation

Perhaps the most unique aspects in clinical bioinformatics as compared with research sequencing is the deep validation that needs to be performed before launching of the clinical assay. In typical NGS guidelines, the bioinformatics component of the validation has not been thoroughly detailed. However, some publications, including the checklists provided by the College of American Pathologists and the recent guidelines specifically on bioinformatics pipelines by the Association of Molecular Pathologists, provide much more detail into how to think about assay validation in terms of the bioinformatics components.[23–25]

For typical clinical assays, sensitivity and specificity are common metrics to analyze during validation. However, in sequencing assays, most positions are not expected to have a variant and, thus, sensitivity is less meaningful. Laboratories therefore often think about sensitivity and positive predictive value. Determining these values for the sequencing assay can be difficult. The recent Association of Molecular Pathologists guidelines suggest at least 59 variants tested per variant type (SNV, small indel, large indel, complex variant, etc). Although this strategy is useful for challenging variants, in practice it may be underpowered to evaluate true sensitivity and positive predictive value. However, there are resources to help the laboratory reach the required number of variants, including the following.

- NIST Genome in a Bottle—A series of very well-characterized genomes that have been sequenced across multiple technologies to be used for comparison purposes. Corresponding samples are also available.[26]
- Illumina Platinum Genomes—High-coverage genome sequencing of 17 members from a CEPH family.[27]
- The Centers for Disease Control and Prevention's Get-RM program—Includes regions orthogonally validated by external laboratories, including a detailed pharmacogenomic characterization of 137 samples.[28,29]
- Synthetic cell lines—Provided by a variety of vendors, these samples are engineered to contain multiple variants in 1 sample and, thus, can be good to test a high number of variants in a single run

---

Box 5
Orthogonal Confirmation of Genomic Variants

Typically, especially in germline molecular genetics, reported variants identified by genomic sequencing are confirmed by an orthogonal method. However, this can cause both increased costs and a delayed turn-around time, specifically in exome and genome sequencing where the primer pairs may need to be developed on the fly. To minimize this occurrence, some laboratories have implemented policies to not confirm variants based on classes (ie, likely benign and benign variants, or carrier status variants). With the high accuracy of most next-generation sequencing data (excluding the difficult regions discussed in **Box 2**), it may not be necessary to do this for every variant.

Indeed, some laboratories have shown high enough accuracy to either reduce or eliminate confirmation with Sanger sequencing of the identified single nucleotide variants and indels.[1,39–41] Although these publications did not contain many false-positive calls on which to set their metrics, they did show that the general framework exists. Confirmation of low-quality calls or calls in difficult regions may still be necessary, but using specific metrics to identify only high-quality true positives that do not need confirmation will add a direct benefit to the laboratory, providers, and patients.

- In silico–derived variation—There are numerous tools that take raw sequence data and use in silico algorithms to insert variation into the sample.[30–32] These tools can serve as a good proxy for difficult variation, but should not supplement actual samples.

These datasets, as well as internal and external samples with known variation, can help the laboratory to properly set thresholds for determining false-positive calls. Similarly, these samples can help the laboratory to determine the threshold for high-confidence true positives, that is, variants that may not need orthogonal confirmation. For further detail, see **Box 5**.

In addition to sensitivity and positive predictive value, it is important for the laboratory to properly version each pipeline and to capture the exact pipeline through which a specific sample was run. Changes to the pipeline need to be revalidated. The scope of revalidation should coincide with the scope of the changes. For instance, a new variant calling pipeline should dictate a complete revalidation, whereas updating an interpretation database may just require a simple equivalency check. It is up to the molecular geneticist/pathologist to determine the scope of revalidation and, thus, is a further reason why a thorough understanding of the process is required.

Infrastructure and Storage Policy

The discussion of bioinformatics in clinical genomic sequencing is incomplete without a basic understanding of information infrastructure and current computing paradigms used to plan and manage infrastructure for computation and analysis of vast amount of NGS data. This field is fast evolving, but there are 3 general approaches a laboratory or an organization can take.

- On Premises—This is the traditional way of implementing information and computing infrastructure. This strategy usually is a combination of HPC and grid computing implementation with analysis and bioinformatics pipeline software installed and implemented within an organization's firewall.
- Cloud—This technology is an emerging way of doing large-scale computation and analysis without spending unnecessary amounts of money and time on infrastructure outright. It is usually the way smaller organizations and startups implement their infrastructure.
- Hybrid—Most large organizations tend to lean toward hybrid approach, which is a combination of both approaches mentioned, mostly owing to various regulatory and systems requirements and considerations.

As with the need for infrastructure plan, there is a need to create policies that take systems view of bioinformatics data to ensure the bioinformatics processes run with efficiency, optimizing data processing and storage, and in adherence to regulatory requirements. **Box 6** goes over some common topics to consider for data policy implementation.

FUTURE DIRECTIONS

Genome-scale sequencing is on the cusp of being the routine assay for not only diagnostics, but also for the screening of healthy individuals and even newborns. There are numerous advances in algorithms, technology, and computation that will enable faster, more accurate, and more complete genomic sequencing. These advances include the following.

Box 6
Common Topics to Consider for Data Policy Implementation

Some important topics to consider while planning for implementation of data policy for an organization or a research group include data format used, data compression, metadata, storage, backup, Intellectual Property/Patient Health Information, data life cycle, and retention periods, in addition to data organization and data quality assurance. Setting best practices to be followed by the bioinformatics team is critical here, to be able to track and maintain original and reported data and to keep storage costs within budget. Another critical aspect of clinical bioinformatics is maintaining data security. This goal can be achieved by implementing measures to ensure data integrity, for instance, by appropriately understanding roles, ownership, and end users of clinical data. Similarly, the data policy needs to adhere to regulatory considerations, such as the Health Insurance Portability and Accountability Act, Clinical Laboratory Improvement Amendments, and state regulations, that an organization's data may fall under. It is good practice in next-generation sequencing data management to have regular data audits with the team to ensure that best practices and data policy items are implemented. Designing and implementing these policies upfront is critical to the long-term success of the organization, including designing a data architecture and integration platform that is not just for current needs but flexible enough to handle future challenges.

- Longer read sequencing that will enable better resolution of the genome and more accurate alignment.
- GPU-based software that will enable increased parallelization and faster computation.
- A graph-based reference genome that will enable a true complete genome path and more accurate alignment, especially for underrepresented ethnicities.

Genomic sequencing is also starting to make use of general advances in computation, specifically around big data. There are already examples of using machine learning approaches in variant calling [33] and similar machine learning and natural language processing approaches will be able to increase the accuracy of variant interpretation as well. There is also promising work extending the laboratory beyond its silo and better integrating laboratory findings with deep mining of clinical data and patient phenotypes. This data integration will also enable interpretation of the full genome, without being limited to the coding regions, which are the main focus of current clinical interpretation workflows. Taken together, these advances will help to unleash the potential of an individual's genome within the continuum of clinical practice.

SUMMARY

Genomic sequencing is increasingly becoming part of clinical practice and the size and scope of the data generated relies more and more heavily on bioinformatics. Although the underlying algorithms and pipelines may seem complex, it is crucial for the molecular geneticist/pathologist to have a thorough understanding of the bioinformatics tools' purpose, outputs, and main underlying assumptions. This understanding includes each of the steps in the process, important quality control metrics and criteria, and validation approaches. Having a broad knowledge of the clinical bioinformatics process can enable the molecular geneticist/pathologist to ensure that the genomic assay is complete, robust, and accurate for clinical practice.

REFERENCES

1. Baudhuin LM, Lagerstedt SA, Klee EW, et al. Confirming variants in next-generation sequencing panel testing by sanger sequencing. J Mol Diagn 2015; 17:456–61.
2. Mason-Suares H, Landry L, Lebo MS. Detecting copy number variation via next generation technology. Curr Genet Med Rep 2016;4:74–85.
3. den Dunnen JT, Dalgleish R, Maglott DR, et al. HGVS recommendations for the description of sequence variants: 2016 update. Hum Mutat 2016;37:564–9.
4. Lek M, Karczewski KJ, Minikel EV, et al. Analysis of protein-coding genetic variation in 60,706 humans. Nature 2016;536:285–91.
5. 1000 Genomes Project Consortium, Auton A, Brooks LD, Durbin RM, et al. A global reference for human genetic variation. Nature 2015;526:68–74.
6. gnomAD browser. Available at: http://gnomad.broadinstitute.org/. Accessed April 16, 2018.
7. Schwarz JM, Rödelsperger C, Schuelke M, et al. MutationTaster evaluates disease-causing potential of sequence alterations. Nat Methods 2010;7:575–6.
8. Reva B, Antipin Y, Sander C. Predicting the functional impact of protein mutations: application to cancer genomics. Nucleic Acids Res 2011;39:e118.
9. Adzhubei I, Jordan DM, Sunyaev SR. Predicting functional effect of human missense mutations using PolyPhen-2. Curr Protoc Hum Genet 2013;Chapter 7: Unit7.20.
10. Ioannidis NM, Rothstein JH, Pejaver V, et al. REVEL: an ensemble method for predicting the pathogenicity of rare missense variants. Am J Hum Genet 2016;99: 877–85.
11. Wang K, Li M, Hakonarson H. ANNOVAR: functional annotation of genetic variants from high-throughput sequencing data. Nucleic Acids Res 2010;38:e164.
12. McLaren W, Gil L, Hunt SE, et al. The ensemble variant effect predictor. Genome Biol 2016;17:122.
13. Cingolani P, Platts A, Wang le L, et al. A program for annotating and predicting the effects of single nucleotide polymorphisms, SnpEff: SNPs in the genome of Drosophila melanogaster strain w1118; iso-2; iso-3. Fly (Austin) 2012;6:80–92.
14. Ramos AH, Lichtenstein L, Gupta M, et al. Oncotator: cancer variant annotation tool. Hum Mutat 2015;36:E2423–9.
15. Liu X, White S, Peng B, et al. WGSA: an annotation pipeline for human genome sequencing studies. J Med Genet 2016;53:111–2.
16. Strande NT, Riggs ER, Buchanan AH, et al. Evaluating the clinical validity of gene-disease associations: an evidence-based framework developed by the clinical genome resource. Am J Hum Genet 2017;100:895–906.
17. Samocha KE, Robinson EB, Sanders SJ, et al. A framework for the interpretation of de novo mutation in human disease. Nat Genet 2014;46:944–50.
18. Petrovski S, Wang Q, Heinzen EL, et al. Genic intolerance to functional variation and the interpretation of personal genomes. PLoS Genet 2013;9:e1003709.
19. Landrum MJ, Lee JM, Benson M, et al. ClinVar: improving access to variant interpretations and supporting evidence. Nucleic Acids Res 2017;46:D1062–7.
20. Li MM, Datto M, Duncavage EJ, et al. Standards and guidelines for the interpretation and reporting of sequence variants in cancer: a joint consensus recommendation of the association for molecular pathology, American Society of Clinical Oncology, and College of American Pathologists. J Mol Diagn 2017; 19:4–23.

21. Richards S, Aziz N, Bale S, et al. Standards and guidelines for the interpretation of sequence variants: a joint consensus recommendation of the American College of Medical Genetics and Genomics and the Association for Molecular Pathology. Genet Med 2015;17:405–24.

22. Yohe SL, Carter AB, Pfeifer JD, et al. Standards for clinical grade genomic databases. Arch Pathol Lab Med 2015;139:1400–12.

23. Roy S, Coldren C, Karunamurthy A, et al. Standards and guidelines for validating next-generation sequencing bioinformatics pipelines: a joint recommendation of the association for molecular pathology and the College of American Pathologists. J Mol Diagn 2018;20:4–27.

24. Aziz N, Zhao Q, Bry L, et al. College of American Pathologists' laboratory standards for next-generation sequencing clinical tests. Arch Pathol Lab Med 2015;139(4):481–93. Available at: https://www.ncbi.nlm.nih.gov/pubmed/25152313. Accessed April 16, 2018.

25. College of American Pathologists (CAP). Accreditation checklists. Available at: http://www.cap.org/web/home/lab/accreditation/accreditation-checklists. Accessed April 16, 2018.

26. Zook JM, Catoe D, McDaniel J, et al. Extensive sequencing of seven human genomes to characterize benchmark reference materials. Sci Data 2016;3:160025.

27. Eberle MA, Fritzilas E, Krusche P, et al. A reference data set of 5.4 million phased human variants validated by genetic inheritance from sequencing a three-generation 17-member pedigree. Genome Res 2017;27:157–64.

28. Pratt VM, Everts RE, Aggarwal P, et al. Characterization of 137 genomic DNA reference materials for 28 pharmacogenetic genes: a GeT-RM collaborative project. J Mol Diagn 2016;18:109–23.

29. Genetic Testing Reference Materials Coordination Program (GeT-RM) - Home. Available at: https://wwwn.cdc.gov/clia/Resources/GetRM/. Accessed April 16, 2018.

30. Duncavage EJ, Abel HJ, Merker JD, et al. A model study of in silico proficiency testing for clinical next-generation sequencing. Arch Pathol Lab Med 2016;140:1085–91.

31. Duncavage EJ, Abel HJ, Pfeifer JD. In silico proficiency testing for clinical next-generation sequencing. J Mol Diagn 2017;19:35–42.

32. Escalona M, Rocha S, Posada D. A comparison of tools for the simulation of genomic next-generation sequencing data. Nat Rev Genet 2016;17:459–69.

33. Poplin R, Newburger D, Dijamco J. Creating a universal SNP and small indel variant caller with deep neural networks. bioRxiv 2016. https://doi.org/10.1101/092890.

34. Zhao H, Sun Z, Wang J, et al. CrossMap: a versatile tool for coordinate conversion between genome assemblies. Bioinformatics 2014;30:1006–7.

35. Lift genome annotations. Available at: http://genome.ucsc.edu/cgi-bin/hgLiftOver. Accessed April 17, 2018.

36. Coordinate remapping service: NCBI. Available at: https://www.ncbi.nlm.nih.gov/genome/tools/remap. Accessed April 17, 2018.

37. ga4gh. ga4gh/benchmarking-tools. GitHub. Available at: https://github.com/ga4gh/benchmarking-tools. Accessed April 16, 2018.

38. Mandelker D, Schmidt RJ, Ankala A, et al. Navigating highly homologous genes in a molecular diagnostic setting: a resource for clinical next-generation sequencing. Genet Med 2016;18:1282–9.

39. Mu W, Lu H-M, Chen J, et al. Sanger confirmation is required to achieve optimal sensitivity and specificity in next-generation sequencing panel testing. J Mol Diagn 2016;18:923–32.

40. Beck TF, Mullikin JC, Biesecker LG, on Behalf of the NISC Comparative Sequencing Program. Systematic evaluation of sanger validation of next-generation sequencing variants. Clin Chem 2016;62:647–54.

41. Strom SP, Lee H, Das K, et al. Assessing the necessity of confirmatory testing for exome-sequencing results in a clinical molecular diagnostic laboratory. Genet Med 2014;16:510–5.

42. Li H, Durbin R. Fast and accurate short read alignment with Burrows-Wheeler transform. Bioinformatics 2009;25:1754–60.

43. Li H, Durbin R. Fast and accurate long-read alignment with Burrows-Wheeler transform. Bioinformatics 2010;26:589–95.

44. NovoAlign | Novocraft. Available at: http://www.novocraft.com/products/novoalign/. Accessed April 16, 2018.

45. Li H. A statistical framework for SNP calling, mutation discovery, association mapping and population genetical parameter estimation from sequencing data. Bioinformatics 2011;27:2987–93.

46. McKenna A, Hanna M, Banks E, et al. The genome analysis toolkit: a MapReduce framework for analyzing next-generation DNA sequencing data. Genome Res 2010;20:1297–303.

47. Poplin R, Ruano-Rubio V, DePristo MA, et al. Scaling accurate genetic variant discovery to tens of thousands of samples. BioRxiv 2017. https://doi.org/10.1101/201178.

48. Erik Garrison, Gabor Marth. Haplotype-based variant detection from short-read sequencing. arXiv, 2012; 1207.3907

49. Ye K, Schulz MH, Long Q, et al. a pattern growth approach to detect break points of large deletions and medium sized insertions from paired-end short reads. Bioinformatics 2009;25:2865–71.

50. Fan X, Abbott TE, Larson D, et al. BreakDancer: identification of genomic structural variation from paired-end read mapping. Curr Protoc Bioinformatics 2014; 45:15.6.1–15.6.11.

51. Handsaker RE, Van Doren V, Berman JR, et al. Large multiallelic copy number variations in humans. Nat Genet 2015;47:296–303.

52. Chen X, Schulz-Trieglaff O, Shaw R, et al. Manta: rapid detection of structural variants and indels for germline and cancer sequencing applications. Bioinformatics 2016;32:1220–2.

53. Fromer M, Purcell SM. Using XHMM software to detect copy number variation in whole-exome sequencing data. Curr Protoc Hum Genet 2014;81:7.23.1-21.

54. Pugh TJ, Amr SS, Bowser MJ, et al. VisCap: inference and visualization of germline copy-number variants from targeted clinical sequencing data. Genet Med 2016;18:712–9.

55. Quinlan AR. BEDTools: the Swiss-army tool for genome feature analysis. Curr Protoc Bioinformatics 2014;47:11.12.1-34.

56. Cleary JG, Braithwaite R, Gaastra K. Comparing variant call files for performance benchmarking of next-generation sequencing variant calling pipelines. bioRxiv 2015. https://doi.org/10.1101/023754.

57. Babraham Bioinformatics - FastQC a quality control tool for high throughput sequence data. Available at: https://www.bioinformatics.babraham.ac.uk/projects/fastqc/. Accessed April 16, 2018.

58. Jun G, Flickinger M, Hetrick KN, et al. Detecting and estimating contamination of human DNA samples in sequencing and array-based genotype data. Am J Hum Genet 2012;91:839–48.

59. Picard Tools - By Broad Institute. Available at: https://broadinstitute.github.io/picard/. Accessed April 16, 2018.

60. Kircher M, Witten DM, Jain P, et al. A general framework for estimating the relative pathogenicity of human genetic variants. Nat Genet 2014;46:310–5.

61. Quang D, Chen Y, Xie X. DANN: a deep learning approach for annotating the pathogenicity of genetic variants. Bioinformatics 2014;31:761–3.

Precision Therapy for Inherited Retinal Disease

At the Forefront of Genomic Medicine

Nicole Koulisis, MD[a,b,c], Aaron Nagiel, MD, PhD[a,b,c],*

KEYWORDS

- Adeno-associated virus (AAV)
- Clustered regularly interspaced short palindromic repeats (CRISPR) • Gene transfer
- Inherited retinal disease • Next-generation sequencing (NGS) • Retinal degeneration
- Sanger sequencing • Subretinal gene therapy

KEY POINTS

- Next-generation sequencing enables rapid and inexpensive whole-genome and exome sequencing. The Sanger method remains vital for variant confirmation and deep intronic sequencing.
- The retina is ideal for gene therapy because it is accessible, is relatively immune privileged, requires only small volumes of medicine, and has measurable anatomic and functional endpoints.
- Food and Drug Administration approval of voretigene neparvovec-rzyl (Luxturna) represents a landmark in the field, with this gene therapy now being delivered at several centers in the United States.
- A rapidly expanding number of gene therapy trials are under way for patients with achromatopsia (CNGA3 and CNGB3), choroideremia (CHM), Stargardt disease (ABCA4), retinitis pigmentosa (RPGR, MERTK, and PDE6B), Usher syndrome (MYO7A), and X-linked retinoschisis (RS1).
- Novel gene targeting techniques, such as clustered regularly interspaced short palindromic repeats (CRISPR)/Cas9, antisense oligonucleotides, and optogenetics also are being employed.

INTRODUCTION

Inherited retinal diseases (IRDs) are a genotypically and phenotypically heterogenous group of disorders affecting the retina. The neurosensory retina is a thin, multilayered structure lining the inner wall of the eye, composed of an intricate network of cells,

[a] Department of Surgery, The Vision Center, Children's Hospital Los Angeles, Los Angeles, CA, USA; [b] The Saban Research Institute, Children's Hospital Los Angeles, Los Angeles, CA, USA; [c] USC Roski Eye Institute, Keck School of Medicine, University of Southern California, 1450 San Pablo Street, Los Angeles, CA 90033, USA
* Corresponding author. 4650 Sunset Boulevard MS#88, Los Angeles, CA 90027.
E-mail address: anagiel@chla.usc.edu

Clin Lab Med 40 (2020) 189–204
https://doi.org/10.1016/j.cll.2020.02.007
0272-2712/20/© 2020 Elsevier Inc. All rights reserved.

labmed.theclinics.com

including photoreceptors, bipolar cells, retinal ganglion cells, and various interneuron subtypes responsible for transducing light stimuli into electrical signals. The peripheral retina is rich in rod photoreceptors, which are important for peripheral vision and low-light vision. In contrast, the macula, whose central 1.5-mm diameter area is known as the fovea, is rich in cone photoreceptors, which are important for high spatial acuity and color vision processing.[1]

Light travels through the full thickness of the retina to the photoreceptor cells, whose outer segments are the site of visual transduction. Essential to the function of these photoreceptors is a monolayer of support cells adjacent to the outer segments, known as the retinal pigment epithelium (RPE).[1] The pathophysiology of many IRDs is believed to arise from dysfunction or loss of the RPE, rod photoreceptors, and/or cone photoreceptors.

IRDs represent a significant source of visual impairment in all age ranges and are thought to affect 200,000 individuals in the United States.[2] These disorders typically affect the retina bilaterally and symmetrically, and syndromic forms may have associated systemic findings, such as sensorineural deafness, nephropathy, neurologic impairment, and other findings. The clinical diagnosis typically is made by clinical examination with adjunct diagnostic testing, which includes optical coherence tomography (OCT), fundus autofluorescence, electroretinography (ERG), and visual field testing. Given the heterogenous genetic nature of IRDs and the extreme specificity of the current treatment modalities, however, genetic testing has become an essential element of diagnosis.[3]

MOLECULAR DIAGNOSTIC TESTING FOR RETINAL DYSTROPHIES

The development of next-generation sequencing (NGS) has changed the field of molecular diagnostics by enabling rapid, high-throughput, whole-genome and whole-exome sequencing at significantly lower costs. Using this technology, targeted panels of known retinal dystrophy genes and candidate genes can be performed at many institutions and commercial laboratories.[4] This technology has greatly improved the diagnostic yield and accuracy of testing, but traditional Sanger sequencing continues to play a role in confirming mutations and for sequencing of deep intronic mutations (eg, CEP290) and guanine-cytosine nucleotide-rich areas (eg, RPGR), which are poorly read by NGS. The field has come a long way since the first IRD gene was reported in 1984 in relation to X-linked retinitis pigmentosa (RP).[5] Since then, there has been a steady rise in the number of genes identified ,with 271 genes linked to IRDs as of 2019 (**Fig. 1**).[6]

NGS not only has facilitated the identification of causative retinal disease genes but also now serves to identify candidates for gene therapy. This is a reflection of significant genetic heterogeneity among patients with IRDs, the difficulty of phenotype-genotype correlation for many conditions (**Fig. 2**), and the need for diagnostic certainty prior to proceeding with gene therapy. Given the risks of bilateral gene therapy surgery, the establishment of a sound genetic diagnosis is crucial and must be supported by segregation analysis, up-to-date variant databases and prediction algorithms, and in some cases in vitro verification of mutational pathogenicity.[7]

GENE THERAPY FOR RETINAL DYSTROPHIES

Over the past 2 decades, a dramatic explosion in understanding of retinal dystrophies, vitreoretinal surgical techniques, and viral vectors[8–10] has created fertile ground for addressing these diseases with gene replacement and other allele-targeting strategies. In most cases, the goal is gene replacement, using a normal copy of the diseased

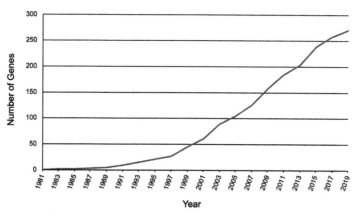

Fig. 1. Number of retinal disease genes identified over the past 38 years. Since the first IRD gene was reported in 1984, there has been a dramatic rise in the number of IRD-related genes identified. As of 2019, 271 genes have been discovered.

gene. Other strategies involve targeting diseased alleles with mutation-specific or exon-specific antisense oligonucleotides.

Viral Vectors for the Retina

To date, several viral vectors, including lentivirus, adenovirus, and adeno-associated virus (AAV), have been explored for use in gene therapy (**Table 1**). Advantages of the lentivirus vector include its large complementary DNA (cDNA) packing capacity (8–10 kilobases [kb]) and its ability to efficiently transduce RPE cells. Disadvantages include its less effective ability to target differentiated photoreceptors and its risk for insertional mutagenesis as it integrates into the target cell's genome.[11] AAV has overwhelmingly become the viral vector of choice for ocular gene delivery, despite its smaller packaging capacity (4.8 kb). This recombinant, nonenveloped, single-stranded, DNA parvovirus has a favorable immunogenicity and toxicity profile, and, by modifying the viral capsid and promoter region, it can be targeted to express protein in specific cell types of the retina.[12] Use of adenovirus has been limited due to its high immunogenicity.

The Retina as a Target for Gene Therapy

The retina offers several advantages for gene therapy.[12] First, the relative immune-privileged status of the subretinal space minimizes host response to viral vector.[13] Second, intravitreal and especially subretinal delivery approaches require a relatively small volume of vector in contrast to systemic delivery.[14] Third, the anatomic accessibility of the retina allows for a direct view of the target tissue during vector delivery and enables noninvasive, multimodal, functional, and anatomic monitoring of the delivery site in an outpatient setting. Finally, given the relatively symmetric nature of disease progression in IRDs, the contralateral eye can serve as a control when assessing safety and efficacy.[15]

Surgical Techniques for Vector Delivery

Intravitreal and subretinal injections are the main techniques for gene therapy delivery for retinal dystrophies. The intravitreal approach is the most straightforward because it requires only topical anesthesia and is routinely performed in the outpatient setting for

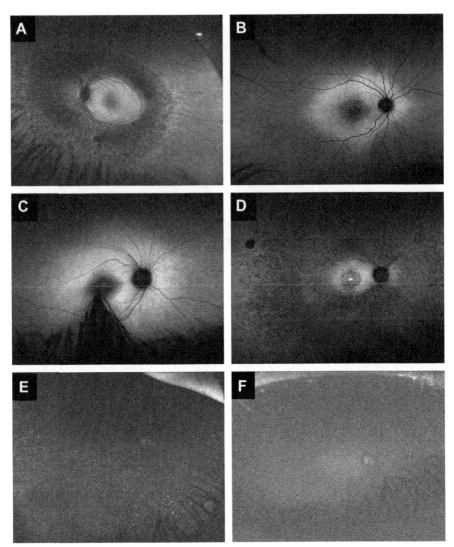

Fig. 2. A sampling of autofluorescence photographs demonstrating the diversity of retinal phenotypes and genotypes. Note that only 1 eye of each patient was included, but that the fellow eye had highly symmetric findings. (*A*) The left eye of a 10-year-old boy with enhanced S-cone syndrome (*NR2E3* c.119-2A > C and c.1142 T > G) features hypoautofluorescence around the vascular arcades. (*B*) In contrast, the right eye of a 6-year-old girl with Stargardt disease (*ABCA4* c.6146delA and c.2424 C > G) demonstrates central hypoautofluorescence with surrounding hyperautofluorescence. (*C*) A similar autofluorescence pattern is seen in an 8-year-old boy with Bardet-Biedl syndrome type 6 (BBS6 c.110 A > G and c.415 C > T). (*D*) In contrast, a 14-year-old girl with Bardet-Biedl syndrome type 1 has marked peripheral hypoautofluorescence and central hyperautofluoresence (*BBS1* c.1169 T > G and c.1181-9C > G). The patients in (*C*) and (*D*) both had associated systemic findings, including polydactyly, cognitive impairment, and truncal obesity. Autofluorescence of LCA associated with (*E*) the *CRB1* gene (homozygous c.2501 G > A) and (*F*) the *RPE65* gene (homozygous c.917 C > A) .

Table 1
Comparison of viral vectors for retinal gene therapy

Vector Type	Genome	Packaging Capacity	Integrates into Target Cell Genome	Infects Dividing and Nondividing Cells	Retinal Cell Targets	Immune Response	Relative Viral Titers	Relative Transduction Efficiency
AAV	4.8 kb (ssDNA)	4.7 kb	No	Yes	RPE, Müller, PRs, GCs	Very low	Moderate	Moderate
Lentivirus	9 kb (ssRNA)	8.0–10.0 kb	Yes	Yes	RPEs > PRs	Low	Moderate	Moderate
Adenovirus	36 kb (dsDNA)	7.5 kb	No	Yes	RPE, Muller	High	High	High

Abbreviations: ds, double-stranded; GCs, ganglion cells; Müller, Müller cells; PRs, photoreceptors; ss, single-stranded.

other indications. There are concerns, however, with accessibility of the vector to photoreceptors and RPE as well as issues with inflammation. Therefore, most trials currently utilize subretinal delivery via pars plana vitrectomy. This approach is familiar to most surgeons but poses a small risk of cataract and retinal detachment. Surgical techniques for subretinal delivery have been optimized and refined.[16] Instrumentation, such as the MicroDose Injection Kit (MedOne Surgical, Sarasota, Florida), allows for pedal-controlled delivery of the viral vector to the subretinal space rather than reliance on manual delivery via an assistant. Intraoperative OCT has become a valuable tool by permitting real-time bleb visualization to ensure subretinal location and monitoring of the fovea to minimize stretch (**Fig. 3**).[17] Novel approaches include ab externo subretinal injection via the suprachoroidal space, which is advantageous in that no vitrectomy or retinotomy are required.[18]

Voretigene Neparvovec-rzyl: Paving the Way

The landmark results of the gene therapy trial for *RPE65*-mediated Leber congenital amaurosis (LCA) led to the US Food and Drug Administration (FDA) approval of voretigene neparvovec-rzyl (Luxturna; Spark Therapeutics, Philadelphia, Pennsylvania) in December 2017. Voretigene neparvovec-rzyl represents the first FDA-approved gene replacement for a hereditary condition and resulted from almost 3 decades of research spearheaded by Jean Bennett, Albert Maguire, Michael Redmond, and many others. Sixteen years after demonstrating efficacy in a canine model,[19] Russell and colleagues[20] published the results of their phase III clinical trial (NCT00999609) in 2017, which showed that treated participants demonstrated significantly improved light sensitivity, visual fields, and ability to navigate in low-light conditions. These statistically significant changes were apparent at 30 days and persisted at 1 year and 4 years after treatment.[21]

Currently, voretigene neparvovec-rzyl gene therapy is performed by selected vitreoretinal surgeons at nine institutions across the United States. The treatment is

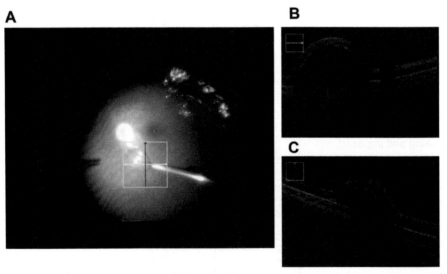

A **B** **C**

Fig. 3. Use of intraoperative OCT during voretigene neparvovec-rzyl delivery. (*A*) Surgical view during delivery of voretigene subretinally with a 38-gauge tip cannula. The live 2-line cross-hair OCT images (horizontal, B; vertical, C) are displayed on the surgical microscope, providing confirmation of subretinal delivery.

performed via vitrectomy followed by subretinal injection of 1.5×10^{11} vector genomes of voretigene neparvovec-rzyl, delivered to the subretinal space in a total volume of 0.3 mL. Typically, the injection site is along the superotemporal vascular arcade at least 2 mm away from the fovea. At this time, the medication costs approximately $425,000 per eye in the United States and will be available in Europe shortly.

Current Retinal Gene Augmentation Trials

Gene therapy for *RPE65*-mediated LCA is a reality, but clinical trials for other retinal dystrophies are moving forward at a rapid pace. To date, there are 27 clinical trials under way using precise gene-specific or allele-specific approaches to treat these conditions (**Table 2**).

Achromatopsia (CNGA3 and CNGB3)

Achromatopsia is a cone dystrophy characterized by severe hemeralopia (day blindness), severe color blindness, and reduced visual acuity.[22] There currently are 6 genes implicated in achromatopsia: *CNGA3*, *CNGB3*, *GNAT2*, *PDE6C*, *PDE6H*, and *ATF6*, of which *CNGB3* and *CNGA3* mutations account for 50% and 25% of all cases, respectively.[23,24] Currently, 5 phase I/II clinical trials are under way for gene delivery of *CNGB3* (NCT02599922 and NCT03001310) and *CNGA3* (NCT02935517, NCT03758404, and NCT02610582).

Choroideremia (CHM)

Choroideremia is an X-linked retinal dystrophy characterized by loss of RPE and secondary degeneration of the choriocapillaris and photoreceptors, and manifests with nyctalopia and progressive peripheral field constriction. It primarily affects men and is caused by variants or deletions in the *CHM* gene, which encodes Rab-escort protein 1 (REP1).[25] The 2-year outcomes of the first phase I/II clinical trial for choroideremia (NCT01461213) showed a statistically significant and sustained improvement of visual acuity in treated eyes (median 4.5 letter gain vs 1.5 letter loss; $P = .04$).[26] These outcomes have been confirmed in other trials (NCT02077361,[27] NCT02553135,[28] and NCT02671539[29]), and there are several ongoing or recruiting trials (NCT02341807, NCT02407678, and NCT03507686), including a phase III trial (NCT03496012).

Stargardt Disease (ABCA4)

Autosomal recessive Stargardt disease has a prevalence of 1 in 10,000 and results from mutations in the *ATP-binding cassette, subfamily A, member 4 (ABCA4)* gene.[30] Vision loss ensues early in life, typically before adolescence owing to atrophy of the macular RPE and photoreceptors. Its pathophysiology includes impaired trafficking and impaired clearance of *N*-retinylidene phosphatidylethanolamine (a retinoid intermediate) from the outer segments of rod and cone photoreceptors, which leads to the pathologic accumulation of lipofuscin in the RPE.[31] Gene therapy offers potential for the treatment of Stargardt, but the size of the *ABCA4* gene is too large (6.8 kb) to be packaged in an AAV vector. Using a lentivirus with a larger cDNA capacity, Sanofi has undertaken a phase I/IIa dose escalation safety study of subretinally injected SAR422459 in 27 subjects (NCT01367444) and followed-up with a larger trial with 46 subjects (NCT01736592). This work is ongoing and results have not yet been published.

Retinitis Pigmentosa (RPGR, MERTK, and PDE6B)

RP is a heterogeneous group of retinal dystrophies characterized by progressive degeneration of rod photoreceptors, followed by secondary degeneration of cone

Table 2
Current clinical trials for inherited retinal diseases

Disease	Gene	Phase	Clinical Trial	Viral Vector/Drug	Sponsor	Mode of Delivery
Achromatopsia	CNGA3	I/II	NCT02935517	rAAV2tYF-PR1.7-hCNGA3	Applied Genetic Technologies Corporation	Subretinal
	CNGA3	I/II	NCT03758404	AAV2/8-hG1.7p.coCNGA3	MeiraGTx UK II Limited	Subretinal
	CNGA3	I/II	NCT02610582	rAAV8.hCNGA3	STZ Eyetrial	Subretinal
	CNGB3	I/II	NCT02599922	rAAV2tYF-PR1.7-hCNGB3	Applied Genetic Technologies Corporation	Subretinal
	CNGB3	I/II	NCT03001310	AAV2/8-hCARp.hCNGB3	MeiraGTx UK II Limited	Subretinal
Choroideremia	CHM	III	NCT03496012	AAV2.REP1	Biogen/NightstaRx Limited	Subretinal
		II	NCT02407678			
		II	NCT03507686			
		II	NCT02671539			
	CHM	I/II	NCT02341807	AAV2-hCHM	Spark Therapeutics	Subretinal
LCA	RPE65	III	NCT00999609	AAV2-hRPE65 v2 (voretigene neparvovec-rzyl)	Spark Therapeutics	Subretinal
		I/II	NCT01208389			
		I	NCT00516477			
	RPE65	I	NCT00481546	rAAV2-CBSB-hRPE65	University of Pennsylvania	Subretinal
	RPE65	I/II	NCT02781480	AAV2/5-OPTIRPE65	MeiraGTx UK II Limited	Subretinal
	GUCY2D	I/II	NCT03920007	AAV-GUCY2D (SAR439483)	Sanofi	Subretinal
	CEP290(c.2991 +1655A > G)	I/II	NCT03872479	CRISPR/Cas9-IVS26 (AGN-151587)	Allergan	Subretinal
	CEP290(c.2991 +1655A > G)	II/III	NCT03913143	Antisense oligonucleotide to IVS26 pre-mRNA (QR-110)	ProQR Therapeutics	Intravitreal
		I/II	NCT03140969			
		I/II	NCT03913130			

Disease	Gene	Phase	NCT number	Construct	Sponsor	Route
RP	RPGR	II/III	NCT03116113	AAV8-RPGR	Biogen/NightstaRx	Subretinal
	RPGR	I/II	NCT03316560	rAAV2tYF-GRK1-RPGR	Applied Genetic Technologies Corporation	Subretinal
	RPGR	I/II	NCT03252847	AAV2-RPGR	MeiraGTx UK II	Subretinal
	PDE6B	I/II	NCT03328130	AAV2/5-hPDE6B	Horama S.A.	Subretinal
	RLBP1	I/II	NCT03374657	AAV8-RLBP1 (CPK850)	Novartis	Subretinal
	MERTK	I	NCT01482195	rAAV2-VMD2-hMERTK	King Khaled Eye Specialist Hospital	Subretinal
	n/a	I/II	NCT03326336	rAAV2.7m8-CAG-ChrimsonR-tdTomato (GS030-DP)	GenSight Biologics	Intravitreal
	n/a	I/II	NCT02556736	AAV2-channelrhodopsin-2	Allergan	Intravitreal
	RHO(P23H)	I/II	NCT04123626	antisense oligonucleotide to P23H mRNA (QR-1123)	ProQR Therapeutics	Intravitreal
Usher syndrome IB	MYO7A	I/II	NCT02065011	EIAV-CMV-MYO7A (UshStat)	Sanofi	Subretinal
Usher syndrome 2A	USH2A(Exon13)	I/II	NCT03780257	antisense oligonucleotide to USH2A Exon13 pre-mRNA (QR-421A)	ProQR Therapeutics	Intravitreal
Stargardt disease	ABCA4	I/II	NCT01736592	Lentivirus-ABCA4 (SAR422459)	Sanofi	Subretinal
XLRS	RS1	I/II	NCT02317887	AAV8-scRS/IRBPhRS	National Eye Institute	Intravitreal
XLRS	RS1	I/II	NCT02416622	rAAV2tYF-CB-hRS1	Applied Genetic Technologies Corporation	Intravitreal

photoreceptors and RPE cells. Symptoms typically include nyctalopia, progressive peripheral field loss, and, in late states, decreased central visual acuity due to cone photoreceptor degeneration. More than 200 genes and upwards of 3000 mutations have been implicated in RP.[32] Inheritance patterns vary and include autosomal recessive (50%–60% of cases), autosomal dominant (30%–40%), and X-linked recessive (5%–15%).

Mutations in the *retinitis pigmentosa GTPase regulator* (*RPGR*) gene have been identified in more than 70% of X-linked recessive families.[32] Currently, there are 3 clinical trials for *RPGR*-associated RP using three different viral vectors; these include 2 phase I/II clinical trials (NCT03316560, NCT03252847) and 1 phase II/III study (XIRIUS, Biogen/NightStaRx; NCT03116113), whose phase I/II dose escalation study has thus far shown positive preliminary safety and efficacy data, including improved central retinal sensitivity.[33,34] The groundwork for all 3 clinical trials comes in large part from prior work done on codon optimization of the *RPGR* sequence, and experiments in 2 *RPGR* mouse models (*RPGR*-KO and Rd9) that showed improved ERG responses in treated mice at 4 months and 6 months.[35,36]

Gene replacement therapy for *MER proto-oncogene tyrosine kinase* (*MERTK*)-associated RP is another example. Efficacious results were shown in *MERTK* mutant rats (Royal College of Surgeons) who underwent subretinal delivery of the human *MERTK* construct (AAV2-VMD2-hMERTK),[37] as part of the preclinical work for the phase I clinical trial (NCT01482195). Thus far, the preliminary results have shown that the vector generally is well tolerated, and 50% of subjects (3/6) demonstrated measurable improvements in visual acuity, although the effect was lost by 2 years in 2 of 3 patients.[38]

Another phase I/II clinical trial under way for RP utilizes an AAV2 vector for delivery of the *phosphodiesterase 6-beta subunit* (*PDE6B*) gene (NCT03328130). *PDE6B*-mediated RP represent 4% to 5% of all RP cases.[39] In the canine model, AAV2 delivery of the *PDE6B* gene halted rod degeneration at 3.5 years follow-up.[40]

Usher Syndrome Type I (MYO7A)

Usher syndrome is a form of syndromic RP affecting 1 in 25,000 people and characterized by sensory impairment of the visual and the audiovestibular systems.[41] Usher syndrome is a heterogeneous disease with 3 clinical subtypes and 9 associated genes.[42] Usher syndrome 1B is caused by mutations in *MYO7A*, which encodes myosin VIIA, an important protein for ciliary transport between photoreceptor inner and outer segments. Deafness and photoreceptor dysfunction manifest at birth with ensuing retinal degeneration. A phase I/IIa trial by Oxford Biomedica (Oxford, UK) (NCT01505062) is evaluating *MYO7A* gene therapy (UshStat) for patients with Usher syndrome, Type 1B. The size of the transgene that expresses myosin VIIA is too large for the AAV vector; thus, the trial employs a subretinal injection of the gene product using an equine lentiviral-based vector. Four patients have been enrolled with good safety outcomes but final results are still pending.[43]

X-Linked Retinoschisis (RS1)

X-linked retinoschisis (XLRS) is an inherited retinal dystrophy in boys that is caused by mutations in the *retinoschisin 1* (*RS1*) gene and characterized by schisis of the retinal layers leading to impaired synaptic transmission from photoreceptors to bipolar cells.[44] The impetus for clinical trials in humans stems from work done in the murine model, which showed that intravitreal delivery of human *RS1* gene (AAV8-RS1) led to restoration of the retinoschisin peptide in its typical histologic distribution, resolution of schisis cavities, and improved ERG b-wave responses.[45] Two phase I/II dose escalation clinical trials for XLRS have been performed (NCT02317887 and NCT02416622) using intravitreally delivered vector.

In the trial (NCT02317887) led by the National Eye Institute, the vector (AAV8-scRS/IRBPhRS) required topical and/or systemic steroids in all 9 patients due to vector-related inflammation. All visual outcome parameters, including visual acuity, returned to baseline by 18 months.[46] The other clinical trial (NCT02416622), led by Applied Genetic Technologies Corporation (Alachua, Florida), showed similar disappointing results and the trial was terminated. Future work is aimed at optimizing the delivery, dose, and immunosuppressive regimen.[47]

NOVEL GENE THERAPY APPROACHES

In addition to the many gene replacement trials, novel approaches are being employed to achieve mutation-specific or allele-specific targeting. Clustered regularly interspaced short palindromic repeats (CRISPR)-Cas9 is an RNA-guided nuclease technique, which represents an exciting potential avenue for diseases not amenable to traditional gene replacement, such as autosomal dominant conditions.[48] CRISPR-Cas9–mediated DNA breaks can be repaired either through homology-directed repair, allowing for knock-in of DNA sequences, or through nonhomologous end joining, which often results in insertions or deletions of random nucleotides at the site (indels). Thus, it may be possible to not only destroy pathogenic alleles but also to perform CRISPR-mediated gene correction in situ or on patient-derived induced pluripotent stem cells in order to generate gene-corrected differentiated cells (eg, RPE or photoreceptors) for autologous cellular transplantion.[3,49,50]

Editas Medicine (Cambridge, MA), in partnership with Allergan (Dublin, Ireland), announced in July 2019 the initiation of the Brilliance phase I/II clinical trial of subretinal AGN-151587 (NCT03872479) for the treatment of LCA caused by the deep intronic c.2991 + 1655A > G (IVS26) mutation in the CEP290 gene.[51] This represents the first in vivo trial of a CRISPR-based therapy to achieve targeted deletion of a cryptic splice site caused by the IVS26 mutation and restore expression of CEP290 protein.[52] Concerns with this treatment strategy include persistence of Cas9 activity and off-target effects at other genomic loci.[52,53]

Other novel therapies for the treatment of IRDs include the use of antisense oligonucleotides to target aberrant pre–messenger RNAs (pre-mRNAs) implicated in IRDs, thereby modulating mRNA splicing and/or stability in an allele-specific fashion.[54] Rather than use CRISPR methods to delete the CEP290 cryptic splice site, ProQR Therapeutics (Leiden, Netherlands) is assessing the safety and efficacy of intravitreally injected antisense oligonucleotide (QR-110) to suppress the IVS26-associated cryptic splice site (NCT03913143, NCT03140969, and NCT03913130).[55]

Other antisense-based clinical trials illustrate the degree to which precision medicine is being utilized for the treatment of IRDs. An intravitreal antisense oligonucleotide that is mutation-specific is being employed against mutant RHO(P23H) mRNA in patients with dominant RHO-associated RP (NCT04123626; QR-1123). Another example is the use of antisense to induce exon-skipping for Usher Syndrome, Type 2A patients with pathogenic variants in exon 13 (NCT03780257; QR-421A).

THE FUTURE OF THE FIELD

Gene therapy is undergoing rapid evolution and expansion as the number of trials dramatically increases. Nowhere is this more apparent than in the field of retinal dystrophies, with a vibrant synergy between molecular diagnosis and precise surgical delivery. The field has rapidly expanded from traditional gene augmentation approaches to allele-specific or mutation-specific suppression using CRISPR or antisense technology. The widespread use of large panels testing the approximately 271 known genes associated with IRD has allowed seeing the landscape of genetic alterations in each patient, improving diagnostic yield, and mitigating against a false assumption of causality. This is especially important for gene therapy candidates, given the significant risks associated with the treatment. As individualized diagnostic and treatment algorithms continue to be developed, equally important will be early molecular diagnosis to facilitate treatment in a timely fashion before significant cellular degeneration has ensued.[56]

The youngest patient treated with subretinal gene delivery to the authors' knowledge was a 22-month-old girl with LCA at Children's Hospital Los Angeles. It is possible that children as young as 12 months could be treated with gene therapy if molecular diagnosis is established by then. The FDA label for voretigene neparvovec-rzyl recommends, however, against its use in children less than 12 months old because of ongoing retinal cell division, which could dilute the genetic material. In light of this, and the increased surgical complexity in very young infants, this seems a practical and scientifically sound lower limit at this time.

The prevalence of autosomal recessive IRDs is estimated to be 1 in 1380 individuals, with 5.5 million people expected to be affected globally.[57] Based on the current diagnostic yield of panel-based genetic testing in IRDs, 40% to 76% of these patients are expected to receive a genetic diagnosis.[4,58,59] Thus, the anticipated number of patients with IRDs who may undergo gene therapy in the future is substantial.

Advances in surgical delivery to the retina also have been an important driver of this blossoming trend in retinal gene therapy. Since developed by Maguire and others,[60] subretinal delivery seems effective and relatively safe, especially with ongoing improvements in vitreoretinal surgery visualization and instrumentation. Although the intravitreal approach represents an attractive outpatient procedure, the subretinal method currently appears to provide the best access to the photoreceptors and RPE, which are the target cell types for most dystrophies.

It is imperative to mention the growing need for a multidisciplinary, team approach when treating IRD patients. This includes having bioinformaticians and molecular pathologists in close communication with a retina specialist, who is in turn supported by genetic counselors, low vision specialists, operating room staff, and photographers familiar with advanced diagnostic testing, such as microperimetry, full-field scotopic sensitivity threshold testing, and ERG.

ACKNOWLEDGMENTS

This work was supported in part by an unrestricted grant to the Department of Ophthalmology at the USC Keck School of Medicine from Research to Prevent Blindness, New York, NY (AN and NK), the Las Madrinas Endowment in Experimental Therapeutics for Ophthalmology (AN), a Knights Templar Eye Foundation pilot grant (AN), and the Donald E. and Delia B. Baxter Foundation (AN).

DISCLOSURE

A. Nagiel serves as a consultant for REGENXBIO. N. Koulisis has nothing to disclose.

REFERENCES

1. Schachat AP, Wilkinson CP, Hinton DR, et al. Ryan's retina. 5th edition. 2013.
2. Yerxa B. Progress in inherited retinal disease drug discovery and development: a foundation's perspective. Pharm Res 2018;35(11):239.

3. Hafler BP. Clinical progress in inherited retinal degenerations: gene therapy clinical trials and advances in genetic sequencing. Retina 2017;37(3):417–23.

4. Stone EM, Andorf JL, Whitmore SS, et al. Clinically focused molecular investigation of 1000 consecutive families with inherited retinal disease. Ophthalmology 2017;124(9):1314–31.

5. Bhattacharya SS, Wright AF, Clayton JF, et al. Close genetic linkage between X-linked retinitis pigmentosa and a restriction fragment length polymorphism identified by recombinant DNA probe L1.28. Nature 1984;309(5965):253–5.

6. Daiger S. RetNet: summaries of genes and loci causing retinal diseases 2019. Available at: https://sph.uth.edu/retnet/sum-dis.htm#D-graph. Accessed October 29, 2019.

7. Yang U, Gentleman S, Gai X, et al. Utility of in vitro mutagenesis of RPE65 protein for verification of mutational pathogenicity before gene therapy. JAMA Ophthalmol 2019;1–9. https://doi.org/10.1001/jamaophthalmol.2019.3914.

8. Flannery JG, Zolotukhin S, Vaquero MI, et al. Efficient photoreceptor-targeted gene expression in vivo by recombinant adeno-associated virus. Proc Natl Acad Sci U S A 1997;94(13):6916–21.

9. Naldini L, Blomer U, Gage FH, et al. Efficient transfer, integration, and sustained long-term expression of the transgene in adult rat brains injected with a lentiviral vector. Proc Natl Acad Sci U S A 1996;93(21):11382–8.

10. Miyoshi H, Takahashi M, Gage FH, et al. Stable and efficient gene transfer into the retina using an HIV-based lentiviral vector. Proc Natl Acad Sci U S A 1997;94(19): 10319–23.

11. Auricchio A, Kobinger G, Anand V, et al. Exchange of surface proteins impacts on viral vector cellular specificity and transduction characteristics: the retina as a model. Hum Mol Genet 2001;10(26):3075–81.

12. Willett K, Bennett J. Immunology of AAV-mediated gene transfer in the eye. Front Immunol 2013;4:261.

13. Bennett J. Immune response following intraocular delivery of recombinant viral vectors. Gene Ther 2003;10(11):977–82.

14. Stieger K, Lheriteau E, Moullier P, et al. AAV-mediated gene therapy for retinal disorders in large animal models. ILAR J 2009;50(2):206–24.

15. Singh MS, Park SS, Albini TA, et al. Retinal stem cell transplantation: balancing safety and potential. Prog Retin Eye Res 2019;100779. https://doi.org/10.1016/j.preteyeres.2019.100779.

16. Davis JL, Gregori NZ, MacLaren RE, et al. Surgical technique for subretinal gene therapy in humans with inherited retinal degeneration. Retina 2019;39(Suppl 1):S2–8.

17. Gregori NZ, Lam BL, Davis JL. Intraoperative use of microscope-integrated optical coherence tomography for subretinal gene therapy delivery. Retina 2019; 39(Suppl 1):S9–12.

18. Ramsden CM, Powner MB, Carr AJ, et al. Stem cells in retinal regeneration: past, present and future. Development 2013;140(12):2576–85.

19. Acland GM, Aguirre GD, Ray J, et al. Gene therapy restores vision in a canine model of childhood blindness. Nat Genet 2001;28(1):92–5.

20. Russell S, Bennett J, Wellman JA, et al. Efficacy and safety of voretigene neparvovec (AAV2-hRPE65v2) in patients with RPE65-mediated inherited retinal dystrophy: a randomised, controlled, open-label, phase 3 trial. Lancet 2017; 390(10097):849–60.

21. Maguire AM, Russell S, Wellman JA, et al. Efficacy, safety, and durability of voretigene neparvovec-rzyl in RPE65 mutation-associated inherited retinal dystrophy: results of phase 1 and 3 trials. Ophthalmology 2019;126(9):1273–85.

22. Simunovic MP, Moore AT. The cone dystrophies. Eye (Lond) 1998;12(Pt 3b): 553–65.

23. Kohl S, Varsanyi B, Antunes GA, et al. CNGB3 mutations account for 50% of all cases with autosomal recessive achromatopsia. Eur J Hum Genet 2005;13(3): 302–8.

24. Wissinger B, Gamer D, Jagle H, et al. CNGA3 mutations in hereditary cone photoreceptor disorders. Am J Hum Genet 2001;69(4):722–37.

25. Seabra MC, Brown MS, Goldstein JL. Retinal degeneration in choroideremia: deficiency of rab geranylgeranyl transferase. Science 1993;259(5093):377–81.

26. Xue K, Jolly JK, Barnard AR, et al. Beneficial effects on vision in patients undergoing retinal gene therapy for choroideremia. Nat Med 2018;24(10):1507–12.

27. Dimopoulos IS, Hoang SC, Radziwon A, et al. Two-year results after AAV2-mediated gene therapy for choroideremia: the alberta experience. Am J Ophthalmol 2018;193:130–42.

28. Lam BL, Davis JL, Gregori NZ, et al. Choroideremia gene therapy phase 2 clinical trial: 24-month results. Am J Ophthalmol 2019;197:65–73.

29. Fischer MD, Ochakovski GA, Beier B, et al. Efficacy and safety of retinal gene therapy using adeno-associated virus vector for patients with choroideremia: a randomized clinical trial. JAMA Ophthalmol 2019. https://doi.org/10.1001/jamaophthalmol.2019.3278.

30. Gerber S, Rozet JM, van de Pol TJ, et al. Complete exon-intron structure of the retina-specific ATP binding transporter gene (ABCR) allows the identification of novel mutations underlying Stargardt disease. Genomics 1998;48(1):139–42.

31. Zhou J, Kim SR, Westlund BS, et al. Complement activation by bisretinoid constituents of RPE lipofuscin. Invest Ophthalmol Vis Sci 2009;50(3):1392–9.

32. Martinez-Fernandez De La Camara C, Nanda A, Salvetti AP, et al. Gene therapy for the treatment of X-linked retinitis pigmentosa. Expert Opin Orphan Drugs 2018;6(3):167–77.

33. Nightstar announces planned initiation of phase 2/3 expansion study in XIRIUS trial for NSR-RPGR in XLRP and reports Third quarter 2018 financial results. 2018. Available at: https://www.globenewswire.com/news-release/2018/11/13/1650095/0/en/Nightstar-Announces-Planned-Initiation-of-Phase-2-3-Expansion-Study-in-XIRIUS-Trial-for-NSR-RPGR-in-XLRP-and-Reports-Third-Quarter-2018-Financial-Results.html. Accessed November 1, 2019.

34. Biogen announces agreement to acquire Nightstar therapeutics to establish clinical pipeline of gene therapy candidates in Ophthalmology. Accessed November 15, 2019. Available at: https://investors.biogen.com/news-releases/news-release-details/biogen-announces-agreement-acquire-nightstar-therapeutics.

35. Tanimoto N, Muehlfriedel RL, Fischer MD, et al. Vision tests in the mouse: functional phenotyping with electroretinography. Front Biosci (Landmark Ed) 2009; 14:2730–7.

36. Fischer MD, McClements ME, Martinez-Fernandez de la Camara C, et al. Codon-optimized rpgr improves stability and efficacy of AAV8 gene therapy in two mouse models of X-linked retinitis pigmentosa. Mol Ther 2017;25(8):1854–65.

37. Conlon TJ, Deng WT, Erger K, et al. Preclinical potency and safety studies of an AAV2-mediated gene therapy vector for the treatment of MERTK associated retinitis pigmentosa. Hum Gene Ther Clin Dev 2013;24(1):23–8.

38. Ghazi NG, Abboud EB, Nowilaty SR, et al. Treatment of retinitis pigmentosa due to MERTK mutations by ocular subretinal injection of adeno-associated virus gene vector: results of a phase I trial. Hum Genet 2016;135(3):327–43.

39. Ferrari S, Di Iorio E, Barbaro V, et al. Retinitis pigmentosa: genes and disease mechanisms. Curr Genomics 2011;12(4):238–49.

40. Pichard V, Provost N, Mendes-Madeira A, et al. AAV-mediated gene therapy halts retinal degeneration in PDE6beta-deficient dogs. Mol Ther 2016;24(5):867–76.

41. Spandau UH, Rohrschneider K. Prevalence and geographical distribution of Usher syndrome in Germany. Graefes Arch Clin Exp Ophthalmol 2002;240(6): 495–8.

42. Tsang SH, Aycinena ARP, Sharma T. Ciliopathy: Usher Syndrome. Adv Exp Med Biol. 2018;1085:167–70.

43. Weleber RG, Stout T, Lauer AK, et al. Early findings in a Phase I/IIa clinical program for Usher syndrome 1B (USH1B; MIM #276900). Invest Ophthalmol Vis Sci 2015;56(7):2286.

44. Wood EH, Lertjirachai I, Ghiam BK, et al. The natural history of congenital X-linked retinoschisis and conversion between phenotypes over time. Ophthalmol Retina 2019;3(1):77–82.

45. Ou J, Vijayasarathy C, Ziccardi L, et al. Synaptic pathology and therapeutic repair in adult retinoschisis mouse by AAV-RS1 transfer. J Clin Invest 2015;125(7): 2891–903.

46. Cukras C, Wiley HE, Jeffrey BG, et al. Retinal AAV8-RS1 gene therapy for X-linked retinoschisis: initial findings from a phase I/IIa trial by intravitreal delivery. Mol Ther 2018;26(9):2282–94.

47. AGTC. AGTC announces topline interim six-month data from phase 1/2 X-linked retinoschisis clinical study; termination of biogen collaboration. 2018. Available at: http://ir.agtc.com/news-releases/news-release-details/agtc-announces-topline-interim-six-month-data-phase-12-x-linked. Accessed October 30, 2019.

48. Cong L, Ran FA, Cox D, et al. Multiplex genome engineering using CRISPR/Cas systems. Science 2013;339(6121):819–23.

49. Burnight ER, Gupta M, Wiley LA, et al. Using CRISPR-Cas9 to generate gene-corrected autologous iPSCs for the treatment of inherited retinal degeneration. Mol Ther 2017;25(9):1999–2013.

50. Ruan GX, Barry E, Yu D, et al. CRISPR/Cas9-mediated genome editing as a therapeutic approach for leber congenital amaurosis 10. Mol Ther 2017;25(2): 331–41.

51. Allergan and editas medicine initiate the brilliance phase 1/2 clinical trial of AGN-151587 (EDIT-101) for the treatment of LCA10. 2019. Available at: http://ir.editasmedicine.com/news-releases/news-release-details/allergan-and-editas-medicine-initiate-brilliance-phase-12. Accessed November 1, 2019.

52. Maeder ML, Stefanidakis M, Wilson CJ, et al. Development of a gene-editing approach to restore vision loss in Leber congenital amaurosis type 10. Nat Med 2019;25(2):229–33.

53. DiCarlo JE, Mahajan VB, Tsang SH. Gene therapy and genome surgery in the retina. J Clin Invest 2018;128(6):2177–88.

54. Gerard X, Garanto A, Rozet JM, et al. Antisense oligonucleotide therapy for inherited retinal dystrophies. Adv Exp Med Biol 2016;854:517–24.

55. Collin RW, den Hollander AI, van der Velde-Visser SD, et al. Antisense oligonucleotide (AON)-based therapy for leber congenital amaurosis caused by a frequent mutation in CEP290. Mol Ther Nucleic Acids 2012;1:e14.

56. Cideciyan AV, Jacobson SG, Beltran WA, et al. Human retinal gene therapy for Leber congenital amaurosis shows advancing retinal degeneration despite enduring visual improvement. Proc Natl Acad Sci U S A 2013;110(6):E517–25.

57. Hanany M, Rivolta C, Sharon D. Worldwide carrier frequency and genetic prevalence of autosomal recessive inherited retinal diseases. Proc Natl Acad Sci U S A 2020;117(5):2710–6.

58. Jiman OA, Taylor RL, Lenassi E, et al. Diagnostic yield of panel-based genetic testing in syndromic inherited retinal disease. Eur J Hum Genet 2019. https://doi.org/10.1038/s41431-019-0548-5.

59. Patel A, Hayward JD, Tailor V, et al. The oculome panel test: next-generation sequencing to diagnose a diverse range of genetic developmental eye disorders. Ophthalmology 2019;126(6):888–907.

60. Maguire AM, High KA, Auricchio A, et al. Age-dependent effects of RPE65 gene therapy for Leber's congenital amaurosis: a phase 1 dose-escalation trial. Lancet 2009;374(9701):1597–605.

Therapeutic Gene Editing with CRISPR

A Laboratory Medicine Perspective

Elan Hahn, MD[a],*, Matthew Hiemenz, MD, MS[b,c]

KEYWORDS

- Gene editing • CRISPR-Cas • TALEN • Zinc finger nuclease • CAR-T • GUIDE-seq
- CIRCLE-seq • DISCOVER-seq

KEY POINTS

- Therapeutic gene editing with the clustered regularly interspaced short palindromic repeat (CRISPR)–Cas system offers significant improvements in specificity and programmability compared with previous methods.
- CRISPR editing strategies can be used ex vivo and in vivo with many theoretic disease applications.
- Off-target effects of CRISPR-mediated gene editing are an important outcome to be aware of, minimize, and detect.
- The current methods of regulatory approval for personalized therapies are complex and may be proved inefficient as these therapies are implemented more widely.
- The role of pathologists and laboratory medicine practitioners is vital to the clinical implementation of therapeutic gene editing.

THE CURRENT STATE OF THERAPEUTIC GENE EDITING
The Promise of Therapeutic Gene Editing

The sequencing of the human genome represented a revolutionary shift in the understanding of human disease. Since its publishing in the early 2000s there have been remarkable steps made in both constitutional and somatic genetics, elucidating the causes of many developmental and cancer predisposition syndromes, as well as causative mutations in sporadic malignancy. As more is learned about the mechanisms of inheritance and pathogenicity, clinicians become more and more aware of

[a] Department of Laboratory Medicine and Pathobiology, University of Toronto, Medical Sciences Building, Room 6231, 1 King's College Circle, Toronto, Ontario M5S 1A8, Canada; [b] Department of Pathology and Laboratory Medicine, Children's Hospital Los Angeles, Los Angeles, California 90027, USA; [c] Department of Pathology, Keck School of Medicine of USC, Los Angeles, California 90033, USA
* Corresponding author.
E-mail address: elan.hahn@medportal.ca

Clin Lab Med 40 (2020) 205–219
https://doi.org/10.1016/j.cll.2020.02.008
0272-2712/20/© 2020 Elsevier Inc. All rights reserved.

labmed.theclinics.com

the complexity of genomic expression. Remarkably, in that same time, there has been an exponential increase in the efficiency of genomic sequencing and data collection coupled with an exponential decrease in cost.[1]

Genetic disorders account for a large proportion of hospital admissions, morbidity, and mortality, and affect a significant proportion of the population.[2] The advent of whole-genome and whole-exome sequencing and their use in clinical diagnostics has identified many genes with many culprit mutations. At present, clinicians find themselves at a nexus, where sequencing power and efficiency are coinciding with a plethora of genomically well-characterized heritable and somatic diseases. What follows is not only the ability to understand the genomic pathogenicity of certain conditions, provide screening and diagnoses for patients and families, and develop targeted therapies but also the need to repair, or edit, the mutated gene and restore its wild-type function. Genomic editing is a precise way to change the DNA of a cell, using recombinant or bacterial enzymes. Given the prevalence of diseases with genetic bases, the ability to edit genes will have an unparalleled impact on medicine and population health, and, as molecular diagnostics continue to improve, the targets for gene editing will only increase.

The Evolution of CRISPR Gene Editing

The discovery of restriction enzymes was fundamental in the development of the recombinant DNA technologies that would become the cornerstone of gene therapy, including gene editing.[3,4] Although ground breaking, the initial techniques lacked efficiency, with recombination only occurring in 1 of 10^3 to 10^9 cells[5]; specificity for site of recombination, with recombination happening at off-target sites at a high frequency[6]; and feasibility. The discovery of double-stranded breaks (DSBs) was essential in the effort to increase recombinant site specificity, affording a substantial increase in frequency of binding at target sites,[7] as well as indicating that new mutations can be created during the repair of these breaks through a process called nonhomologous end joining (NHEJ).[8] In order to achieve DSB, naturally found meganucleases, endonucleases with larger binding domains, were used. Despite offering increased binding specificity and efficiency, the meganuclease-binding domains were too large to feasibly find matches to all desired binding sites, and NHEJ would possibly repair the DSBs without DNA insertion, or by randomly deleting or adding genetic material to the break site.[9] The development of zinc finger nucleases (ZFNs) helped solve the issue of binding site specificity and flexibility. Zinc fingers are small protein structural motifs, stabilized by at least 1 zinc ion, that are capable of binding to DNA in a site-specific manner, recognizing 3-bp sequences.[10] Multiple zinc fingers can be combined to allow specificity in uniquely recognizing a flexible array of binding sites,[11] and, when fused with the Fok I endonuclease cleavage domain, are able to initiate DSBs.[12] Transcription activator–like effector nucleases (TALENs) were the next strategy in gene editing.[13] TALENs are transcription activator–like effector proteins from *Xanthomonas* spp bacteria that are chimerically fused to Fok I endonucleases and can bind with a site specificity of 1 base.[14] These gene editing strategies, although a vast improvement on previous methods, still fall short of attaining clinically feasible flexibility, programmability, and specificity, especially compared with clustered regularly interspaced short palindromic repeat (CRISPR) gene editing strategies.

CRISPR and adjacent well-conserved genes, CRISPR-associated genes (Cas), were initially studied as they related to bacterial immunity.[15] Bacteria and archaea use the CRISPR-Cas complex to process and store viral DNA for use in the event of future infection; once infected, recognition of viral DNA initiates silencing of the offending pathogen.[16] This stored viral DNA can be transmitted to daughter cells and other bacteria.[17] The repeated segments of CRISPR are separated by nonrepeating, phage-derived segments, termed spacers.[18] The spacers are transcribed into short CRISPR RNAs that guide Cas enzyme activity.[19] Highly conserved sequences called protospacer-adjacent motifs (PAMs) are located within the spacers and are critical for Cas binding of the nontargeted DNA.[20] In the bacterial CRISPR system, 2 short RNAs are required; however, for implementation in gene editing, these were chimerized into a single guide RNA (sgRNA), allowing significant ease of use in subsequent studies and eukaryotic applications.[21–23] The CRISPR-Cas9 complex is used to bind and cleave DNA at a targeted sequence, specified by the programmable sgRNA necessarily upstream of a Cas-specific PAM, and create a double-stranded or single-stranded break.[24] The break is then either repaired randomly (with possible insertions or deletions) by NHEJ, by using a provided template, in homology-directed repair (HDR), or via targeted base editing through deaminase fusion to the Cas9 DNA-binding domain.[24,25] Recent work has shown the ability to predict the repaired sequence.[26] Multiple variations of the CRISPR-Cas system are being developed and used to maximize efficiency in different settings, dictated by the desired outcome and the cell target.[27]

CRISPR GENE EDITING
Ex Vivo Applications of CRISPR

Of the human applications of CRISPR-Cas–mediated gene editing, ex vivo methods are more developed and less technically challenging than the in vivo approaches. Ex vivo gene editing involves removing cells from the patient, performing gene editing on the removed cells, and transplanting them back into the patient.[25] Performing gene editing in the laboratory setting allows more sensitive dosing and more effective delivery, such as electroporation, which uses electrical pulses to create pores in the target cell membranes through which the DNA and/or RNA enters.[28] Ex vivo gene editing has been studied using ZFNs and TALENs for a variety of disease conditions.[29–32] Because of the increased feasibility and efficiency relative to other strategies, as outlined earlier, CRISPR-Cas9 is becoming the preferred method for gene editing, including but not limited to the ex vivo setting, and is being applied to many disease states.[33,34]

Chimeric antigen receptor T-cell therapy

T cells are readily edited in the ex vivo setting for use in cancer immunotherapeutics using chimeric antigen receptor T (CAR-T) cells.[35] In CAR-T therapy, the T cells undergo ex vivo editing to express CARs. These receptors consist of an extracellular antigen-binding domain and an intracellular signaling component. The extracellular component can be engineered to recognize specific cancer antigens, and, once bound, the intracellular signaling component activates the T cell to kill the bound cell.[36] These cells have been used with promising results in the treatment of B-cell leukemia, in particular B acute lymphoblastic leukemia (B-ALL), where the antigen-binding domain of the CAR is targeted against CD (cluster of differentiation) 19.[37] The increased specificity of CRISPR-Cas9 has allowed advancement of CAR-T therapies in the treatment of B-ALL where the CAR can be incorporated into the T-cell receptor α constant (TRAC) locus, as opposed to the conventional random insertion, which is under the control of the endogenous T-cell receptor promoter.[38] These cells show more consistent CAR expression and increased efficacy compared with the conventional strategy.[38] CAR-T–cell therapies have been studied in other malignancies, such as melanoma, with promising results in vitro and in animal models.[39]

Hemoglobinopathies

Genetic diseases affecting hematopoietic stem progenitor cells (HSPCs) provide an efficient target for CRISPR-Cas9 gene editing in humans. These cells can be edited and returned to the patient to then give rise to a lineage of so-called corrected cells. Certain hematologic diseases possess well-characterized genetic abnormalities that are more amenable to CRISPR-Cas9 editing of HSPCs.[40] Sickle cell disease (SCD) is one such condition. SCD is characterized by a single base pair substitution that is responsible for the pathologic protein product, resulting in hemoglobin tetramers that polymerize on deoxygenation causing devastating morbidity and mortality.[41] Initially, editing of HSPCs from patients with SCD was studied using ZFNs and TAL-ENs, but CRISPR-Cas9 was shown to be more efficient in targeting the specific caus-ative point mutation in SCD.[42] The understanding of the molecular genetic mechanism of SCD and other hemoglobinopathies, such as β-thalassemia, has allowed other cre-ative approaches to therapeutic gene editing in these conditions.[43] For example, the gene responsible for silencing fetal hemoglobin can be targeted by the CRISPR-Cas9 system, resulting in production of fetal hemoglobin and alleviation of hemoglobinopathy-related symptoms in SCD.[44] The flow-down effects of HSPC edit-ing coupled with the well-characterized, specific genetic causes and pathophysiol-ogies, make hemoglobinopathies an attractive and effective early target for clinical CRISPR-Cas9–mediated gene editing.

In Vivo Applications of CRISPR

In contrast with ex vivo gene editing, in vivo techniques involve delivery of the CRISPR-Cas elements to the affected cells in their physiologic stations throughout the body. Effectively editing the affected cells in vivo eliminates the need of finding and targeting progenitor cells and/or removing the targeted cells for gene editing, thereby vastly increasing the breadth of disorders that are under the potential scope of therapeutic gene editing.[45] The CRISPR-Cas elements are delivered as plasmid DNA or messenger RNA, or directly as proteins, without any modification or packaging, each with its own advantages and disadvantages.[46–48] These ele-ments can be delivered in several ways, categorized as viral, physical, and chem-ical delivery methods. The choice of delivery method presents a major difficulty with in vivo gene editing, with the goals of controlling the distribution of CRISPR-Cas9 and limiting off-target effects and immunotoxicity in response to viral peptides.[49]

Delivery of CRISPR

Viral delivery methods are able to reliably infect cells of many tissue types regardless of proliferative status, causing little cellular damage and minimal immune response.[50] This ability has made viral vectors the preferred method of CRISPR-Cas9 delivery.[51] The lentiviral vector was initially used but has fallen out of favor because of the muta-genesis and oncogenesis that results from incorporation of the viral DNA into the host genome.[52] Adeno-associated viral (AAV) vectors and adenoviral (AV) vectors have been used increasingly, because of the extrachromosomal, nonincorporating nature of their DNA.[53] In addition, AAV and AV vector delivery methods are less immunogenic than their lentiviral counterparts, with AAV vectors providing the greatest benefit in this regard.[54] The major drawback to AAV and AV vector delivery is the limited packaging size, requiring dual-delivery methods to package the Cas9-encoded DNA, sgRNA, and template DNA.[55] Nonviral delivery methods, including physical and chemical de-livery methods, are being developed to combat the risks of recombinant mutagenesis, immunotoxicity, and limited packaging capacity.[56–58] Physical delivery methods include electroporation and hydrodynamic injection (HDI). Electroporation, as discussed earlier, entails using pulses of electricity to create pores in the cellular membranes, through which the CRISPR-Cas machinery travels.[28] Although this technique has been used in the experimental treatment of retinal diseases, the in vivo utility and scalability are questionable.[59,60] HDI involves injection of a large volume of fluid along with the CRISPR-Cas elements, resulting in cellular uptake because of hydrodynamic pressure.[61] HDI techniques are in their infancy and are limited by circulatory patterns and the lack of clinical applications.[62] Chemical delivery methods include lipids, polymers, and inorganic nanoparticles alone or in combination. Lipid methods use micelles to fuse with the target cell membrane, depositing their contents intracellularly.[63] Cationic polymers are a low-cost alternative that allow control of structure and ease in chemical diversification.[64] The CRISPR-Cas elements are contained within a polymer with specificity for tumor-expressed antigens and/or receptors, and, once arriving in the tumor, can be exposed by enzymatic degradation.[65] Inorganic nanoparticles offer flexibility of size and surface functionalization, which allows control of the rate of uptake without inciting an immune reaction.[66] For example, gold nanoparticles are coated with Cas9 RNP, donor DNA, and an endosomal disruptive polymer.[66] The polymer initiates endocytosis with subsequent disruption of the endosome and exposure of the Cas9 RNP and donor DNA.[66] Gold nanoparticles allow conjugation with both CRISPR-Cas9 machinery and donor DNA at variable sizes while being endocytosed by a variety of cell types.[67] Delivering CRISPR-Cas9 is a growing field with many theoretically applicable new technologies.[68]

CRISPR in retinal diseases and muscular dystrophy

In vivo gene editing has been studied in several disease models, including retinal disease and Duchenne muscular dystrophy (DMD). Many different heritable retinal diseases have been studied in the context of gene editing with CRISPR-Cas9, including retinitis pigmentosa, retinal dystrophy, age-related macular degeneration, and Leber congenital amaurosis.[69] Retinal diseases are readily amenable to in vivo gene editing because of their known genetic bases, immune privilege, and lack of traditional treatments.[70] CRISPR-Cas9 technologies are particularly well suited to retinal diseases because of the small size of the components that are readily deliverable to the retinal cells.[70] Theoretically, HDR-mediated gene editing would be able to edit out mutations; however, because of the postmitotic nature of retinal cells, gene disruption by NHEJ is favored, especially in dominant diseases.[60] For example, mutations in the RHO are the most common cause of inherited retinal diseases, resulting in retinitis pigmentosa.[59] CRISPR-Cas9–mediated RHO knockdown has been studied in mice, with gene knockdown specific to the mutated allele.[71] DMD is caused by mutations in the DMD gene on the X chromosome, responsible for maintaining muscle integrity.[72] These mutations are usually deletions but can be duplications or point mutations that result in frameshifting and early termination of translation, with little to no dystrophin produced.[73] In certain cases, revertant muscle fibers have been discovered, showing secondary mutations correcting the reading frame.[73] CRISPR-Cas9 gene editing methods are a logical strategy to use in patients with DMD with frameshift mutations. In vivo approaches have been used, with promising results in correcting the reading frame in mice, with partial recovery of functional dystrophin protein and improved muscle function observed after systemic infusion.[74–77] In vivo gene editing has been studied in many disease states, with various genetic targets, with different theoretic physiologic bases and varied success. This area of research is growing and has a multitude of applications.

THE LABORATORY MEDICINE PERSPECTIVE
Off-Target Effects

CRISPR-Cas9 strategies for gene editing offer several advantages compared with other methods, as discussed earlier, most importantly increased specificity for binding site.[78] Even with malleable target sequences and increased specificity, CRISPR-Cas9 gene editing is at risk for off-target effects.[79,80] Although the specificity is high, there are few genomic loci not at risk for off-target activity.[81] Off-target gene editing can obscure results in research and clinical settings, in addition to introducing unwanted effects and potential patient harm, including mutagenesis and oncogenesis.[82] As such, multiple strategies have been used to limit off-target effects. Theoretically, only 1 Cas9 complex can occupy the intended site in the genome within each cell, thus limiting the concentration of Cas9 or sgRNA, or both, would limit off-target effects.[79,80,83] Other strategies include developing a preformed Cas9-sgRNA complex that is quickly degraded on entering the cell, thereby decreasing off-target binding.[84] In addition, a Cas9 was engineered such that it requires the presence of a small cell-permeable molecule to become active and begin genome editing, increasing specificity and limiting off-target effects.[85] Other methods, similarly decreasing Cas9 activity, have been studied as well, including reducing the energetics of the Cas9-sgRNA complex-target DNA interaction by changing amino acids within the Cas9 protein.[86,87] Pairing Cas9 nickases, which each create a single-stranded break on different strands of DNA, as opposed to nucleases, which create DSBs, allows a dramatic decrease in off-target effects.[88,89] Using truncated sgRNAs, shorter than the typical 20 nucleotides, has also been found effective in decreasing off-target effects, especially when combined with paired nickases.[90,91] Similarly, modifying the ribose-phosphate backbone of sgRNAs shows reduced off-target activity, perhaps because of the decreased stability with mismatched DNA sequences.[92] With the current strategies and more being developed, researchers are doing their best to limit off-target effects before implementation. The reality is that there will always be some off-target activity, and determining the extent and severity is of paramount importance.

Computational methods

Computational methods have been developed to predict possible off-target loci based on the targeted sequence.[81] These tools can be used to develop primers that would allow sequencing of the potential off-target loci.[81] The ability to computationally generate potential off-target sites is a useful theoretic tool in providing areas in need of posttherapeutic attention. Whole-genome sequencing in the posttherapeutic setting would theoretically identify off-target CRISPR activity; however, the cost and scale that would be required to find low-frequency events in large cell populations make this approach impractical.[93,94] In addition, pretherapeutic whole-genome sequencing can identify patient-specific variants that can provide a personalized list of potential off-target loci.[95] In order to feasibly ascertain the reality of the posttherapeutic setting, targeted validated laboratory approaches to quantify and qualify the landscape of off-target activity are necessary.

GUIDE-seq

One such technology for evaluating off-target activity is termed GUIDE-seq (genome-wide, unbiased identification of double-strand breaks enabled by sequencing).[83,96] In the development of this method, the researchers attempted to remove the bias introduced by the discussed computational, prediction-based methods, which assumes that off-target sites will be similar in sequence to the target site, which is not necessarily the case. GUIDE-seq uses the incorporation of blunt double-stranded oligodeoxynucleotides (dsODNs) at the CRISPR-Cas9–induced DSBs. These dsODNs are sequenced by ligating a single-tailed sequencing adapter to randomly sheared DNA from cells transfected with both dsODNs and CRISPR-Cas9 components. This method allows specific amplification because of the requirement of primers to the dsODNs as well as the single-tailed adapters. The single-tailed nature of the adapters allows unidirectional amplification of each dsODN, providing reads of genomic data on either side of the DSB site. In addition, molecular barcodes were implemented for accurate assessment of unique sequencing reads.

CIRCLE-seq

Methods such as GUIDE-seq that rely on transfection of cells with dsODNs is difficult in certain cell types and different laboratory and clinical settings. To combat the low-sensitivity challenges of transfecting cells, circularization for in vitro reporting of cleavage effects by sequencing (CIRCLE-seq) was developed.[97] Randomly sheared DNA is circularized, with nuclease activity resulting in further DSBs, releasing free DNA ends for sequencing.[98] The enrichment of cleaved DNA reduces the necessary number of sequencing reads for the assay. The cleaved DNA, now linearized, contains both ends of the cleavage site, allowing independent off-target identification and sequencing; this is particularly helpful for areas of the genome with highly variable sequence or for which reference sequence is unreliable. CIRCLE-seq is a cell-free method that directly sequences DSBs; therefore, it does not require any DNA damage repair mechanisms to integrate dsODNs, nor does it require a specific delivery method.

DISCOVER-seq

The previously discussed methods for off-target CRISPR activity use purified DNA and are incapable of in vivo use.[99] Discovery of in situ Cas off-targets and verification by sequencing (DISCOVER-Seq) uses the Mre11-Rad50-Nbs1 (MRN) complex, a eukaryotic protein complex that plays an essential role in the processing of DSBs.[100] Randomly sheared DNA was treated with antibodies specific for MRE11 protein. The DNA was then precipitated, unbound from the antibody, and sequenced. The data were processed using the blunt end finder (BLENDER) custom computation pipeline. This method is applicable to the in vivo setting and can identify DSB sites that may lead to other, difficult-to-detect large-scale deletions and rearrangements.[101] GUIDE-seq relies on integration of dsODNs, which is inefficient and not applicable in vivo, and CIRCLE-seq is highly sensitive but overestimates off-target sites, but DISCOVER-seq provides a means to assess off-target activity in vivo in an efficient procedure, using the physiologic repair protein to identify genuine off-target sites of CRISPR-Cas9 activity. This point is important, because in vivo off-target sites can vary significantly from in vitro–identified candidates.[102]

CRISPR and Surgical Pathology

In addition to the clinical pathology laboratory, the surgical pathology laboratory is likely to play a significant role in the development, implementation, and quality assurance of CRISPR-Cas therapeutic gene editing. Following the trajectory of the field, it is reasonable to think that therapeutic gene editing will be implemented in the germ cell, hereditary, and cancer therapeutic settings. While envisioning the practice of therapeutic gene editing, many things must be considered. First, in the germ cell setting, there are many ethical considerations to be aware of, and any work in this area must be approached with caution. In the treatment of heritable diseases, outcome measures, including off-target effects, must be established. For example, in the treatment of sickle cell anemia, pathologist assessment of peripheral blood and, if indicated, bone marrow should be considered, not only to assess efficacy but to detect unwanted hematologic effects.

The therapeutic algorithm in the CRISPR-Cas9–guided treatment of malignant neoplasms remains an interesting topic to consider. Where will it be relative to the timing of surgery and chemoradiation? How will it be delivered to the tumor? If it is delivered before surgical resection, the surgical pathology laboratory will play a large role in determining treatment response, as is the current standard of practice with preoperative chemotherapy and radiation. Depending on the delivery method used, immunohistochemistry for viral elements, light microscopic identification of colored nanoparticles, or even specimen radiography for nanoparticles could be used to assess targeted therapy. Tumor cells may die on treatment, but it is possible, with repaired genomes, in particular repaired driver mutations, that the once-malignant cells may enter the resting phase and cease progression. Circulatory patterns could be harnessed along with HDI to limit off-target effects compared with parenteral infusion. Other delivery methods could include direct injection of the tumors, which may limit effectiveness, because the CRISPR-Cas9 elements may not come into contact with each tumor cell, as they would if deployed intravascularly. Nanoparticles, specific for tumor-expressed antigens, can be used in combination with the abovementioned strategies, to maximize specificity.

In all patients undergoing therapeutic gene editing, off-target editing will take place. DSBs not only can lead to incorporation of the target sequence at an erroneous genomic location but also can predispose to other, large-scale genomic rearrangements, including deletions, duplications, and translocations. The job of the surgical pathologist in identifying off-target gene editing as the nidus of lesional tissue development would be essential, as would the choice of tissue to target with molecular diagnostics in such cases.

REGULATORY CONSIDERATIONS

The implementation of therapeutic gene editing presents a unique regulatory convergence. Therapy with CRISPR-Cas9 may require a different strategy for each prospective patient with a unique disease-causing variant, and thus would require approval by the overseeing governing body each time it is used. Kim and colleagues[103] outline the current status of obtaining regulatory administrative approval for personalized therapies in discussing their development of milasen, a custom-tailored, or N-of-1, drug used to treat a girl with neuronal ceroid lipofuscinosis 7, a variation of Batten disease. The initial genetic panel identified 1 mutation in the known disease-causing gene *MFSD8*, but a second mutation in a disease-causing gene is needed in order to display the disease phenotype.[104] After obtaining institutional review board approval and consent, the investigators performed trio genome sequencing in search of this second aberration. They discovered an SVA (SINE–VNTR–Alu) retrotransposon in *MFSD8*, which, although intronic, would theoretically lead to missplicing of the gene. The therapeutic approach was to use the understanding of the mutation's mechanics in conjunction with the sequencing data to identify or develop a targeted therapy. An antisense oligonucleotide that works in the treatment of spinal muscular atrophy through targeting missplicing was adapted for the development of personalized therapy for the girl with Batten disease.[105] The researchers developed an antisense oligonucleotide to correct missplicing of *MFSD8* and proved its efficacy in cultured fibroblasts. They did this through a US Food and Drug Administration (FDA) Expanded Access

Investigational New Drug application, the only currently available avenue for expedited approval of drugs.[106]

Under FDA oversight, apart from the Expanded Access Investigational New Drug application, regenerative medical techniques have increased access to expedited approval through the Fast Track Designation, Breakthrough Therapy Designation, Regenerative Medicine Advanced Therapy Designation, Priority Review Designation, and Accelerated Approval programs. This increased access is because the "CBER [Center for Biologics Evaluation and Research] recognizes the importance of regenerative medicine therapies and is committed to helping ensure they are licensed and available to patients with serious conditions as soon as it can be determined they are safe and effective".[107] Based on their interpretation of section 506(g) (8) of the Food, Drug, and Cosmetic Act, the FDA defines regenerative medicine therapies as those "including cell therapies, therapeutic tissue engineering products, human cell and tissue products, and combination products using any such therapies or products, except for those regulated solely under section 361 of the Public Health Service Act (PHS Act) (42 U.S.C. 264) and Title 21 of the Code of Federal Regulations Part 1271 (21 CFR Part 1271)." Accordingly, gene therapy, which would lead to lasting cellular effects, is under the umbrella of regenerative medicine therapies, as are viral vectors, allowing for expedited approval.

Even with expedited pathways for FDA approval, there would likely be therapeutic delay and inefficiency. Under the current requirements, each unique therapy is likely to require separate approval, albeit with options for expedited review. An overarching exemption applying to similar gene editing techniques, similar to what is currently used for the minimal manipulation and homologous use of human cells, tissues, and cellular and tissue-based products,[108] could provide timely and efficient access to these therapies. Once a specific gene editing strategy is proved in a certain clinicogenomic setting, this may preclude the need for unique FDA approval, provided there are sufficient similarities between cases.

As clinicians further explore personalized medicine, the degree of personalization is at odds with administrative approval. Sequencing power and reach are increasing, which will undoubtedly continue to generate N-of-1 patients, each in need of expedited approval. Perhaps shifting the perception of these therapies, from drugs to therapeutic technique, termed molecular surgery, is appropriate. In doing this, once the technique is shown to be effective and safe in treating a certain class of genetic abnormalities, it will be approved and can then be applied on a patient-by-patient basis, efficiently.

SUMMARY

Therapeutic gene editing has great promise for advances in the current paradigm of medicine. As next-generation sequencing techniques continue to evolve, becoming more ubiquitous, efficient, and cost-effective, the existing heritable diseases will continue on the path toward full characterization, and the number of novel diseases with documented genetic causes will continue to increase. This progress will yield an environment ripe for therapeutic gene editing. As these therapies approach the clinic, considerations around efficacy and safety, including the minimization of off-target effects, will be of paramount importance. This efficacy will be optimized in the clinical laboratories through strategic choices of delivery methods and surveillance. Before use on patients, each therapy, individualized in nature, will require approval from the local governing administrative body. This approval may be obtained on a case-by-case basis, as is the case with new drugs, or perhaps an avenue will be established to obtain an overarching exemption to similar therapeutic techniques. On clinical implementation, it will be interesting to see how these therapies are received in the germline setting, how they are optimized in the heritable disease setting, where they fit in the cancer therapeutic pathways, and how the role of pathologists and laboratory medicine professionals will evolve in evaluating their safety and efficacy. The authors envision a world where molecular surgery, potentially guided and monitored by the work of laboratory medicine practitioners, is applied to a variety of specific patient disorders with deep and wide-ranging clinical impact.

CONFLICTS OF INTEREST

The authors have no conflicts of interest to disclose.

REFERENCES

1. Mardis ER. A decade's perspective on DNA sequencing technology. Nature 2011;470(7333):198–203.
2. Gonzaludo N, Belmont JW, Gainullin VG, et al. Estimating the burden and economic impact of pediatric genetic disease. Genet Med 2019;21(8):1781–9.
3. Smith HO, Wilcox KW. A restriction enzyme from Hemophilus influenzae. I. Purification and general properties. J Mol Biol 1970;51(2):379–91.
4. Kelly TJ, Smith HO. A restriction enzyme from Hemophilus influenzae. II. J Mol Biol 1970;51(2):393–409.
5. Capecchi MR. Altering the genome by homologous recombination. Science 1989;244(4910):1288–92.
6. Lin FL, Sperle K, Sternberg N. Recombination in mouse L cells between DNA introduced into cells and homologous chromosomal sequences. Proc Natl Acad Sci U S A 1985;82(5):1391–5.
7. Rudin N, Sugarman E, Haber JE. Genetic and physical analysis of double-strand break repair and recombination in Saccharomyces cerevisiae. Genetics 1989;122(3):519–34.
8. Bibikova M, Golic M, Golic KG, et al. Targeted chromosomal cleavage and mutagenesis in Drosophila using zinc-finger nucleases. Genetics 2002;161(3):1169–75.
9. Jeggo PA. DNA breakage and repair. Adv Genet 1998;38:185–218.
10. Klug A, Rhodes D. Zinc fingers: a novel protein fold for nucleic acid recognition. Cold Spring Harb Symp Quant Biol 1987;52:473–82.
11. Miller JC, Holmes MC, Wang J, et al. An improved zinc-finger nuclease architecture for highly specific genome editing. Nat Biotechnol 2007;25(7):778–85.
12. Porteus MH, Baltimore D. Chimeric nucleases stimulate gene targeting in human cells. Science 2003;300(5620):763.
13. Boch J, Scholze H, Schornack S, et al. Breaking the code of DNA binding specificity of TAL-type III effectors. Science 2009;326(5959):1509–12.
14. Li T, Huang S, Zhao X, et al. Modularly assembled designer TAL effector nucleases for targeted gene knockout and gene replacement in eukaryotes. Nucleic Acids Res 2011;39(14):6315–25.
15. Ishino Y, Shinagawa H, Makino K, et al. Nucleotide sequence of the iap gene, responsible for alkaline phosphatase isozyme conversion in Escherichia coli, and identification of the gene product. J Bacteriol 1987;169(12):5429–33.
16. Wiedenheft B, Sternberg SH, Doudna JA. RNA-guided genetic silencing systems in bacteria and archaea. Nature 2012;482(7385):331–8.

17. Sapranauskas R, Gasiunas G, Fremaux C, et al. The Streptococcus thermophilus CRISPR/Cas system provides immunity in Escherichia coli. Nucleic Acids Res 2011;39(21):9275–82.
18. Mojica FJM, Díez-Villaseñor C, García-Martínez J, et al. Intervening sequences of regularly spaced prokaryotic repeats derive from foreign genetic elements. J Mol Evol 2005;60(2):174–82.
19. Brouns SJJ, Jore MM, Lundgren M, et al. Small CRISPR RNAs guide antiviral defense in prokaryotes. Science 2008;321(5891):960–4.
20. Deveau H, Barrangou R, Garneau JE, et al. Phage response to CRISPR-encoded resistance in Streptococcus thermophilus. J Bacteriol 2008;190(4): 1390–400.
21. Jinek M, Chylinski K, Fonfara I, et al. A programmable dual-RNA-guided DNA endonuclease in adaptive bacterial immunity. Science 2012;337(6096):816–21.
22. Cong L, Ran FA, Cox D, et al. Multiplex genome engineering using CRISPR/Cas systems. Science 2013;339(6121):819–23.
23. Mali P, Yang L, Esvelt KM, et al. RNA-guided human genome engineering via Cas9. Science 2013;339(6121):823–6.
24. Komor AC, Kim YB, Packer MS, et al. Programmable editing of a target base in genomic DNA without double-stranded DNA cleavage. Nature 2016;533(7603): 420–4.
25. Porteus MH. A new class of medicines through DNA editing. N Engl J Med 2019; 380(10):947–59.
26. Allen F, Crepaldi L, Alsinet C, et al. Predicting the mutations generated by repair of Cas9-induced double-strand breaks. Nat Biotechnol 2019;37(1):64–72.
27. Cox DBT, Gootenberg JS, Abudayyeh OO, et al. RNA editing with CRISPR-Cas13. Science 2017;358(6366):1019–27.
28. Kaneko T, Sakuma T, Yamamoto T, et al. Simple knockout by electroporation of engineered endonucleases into intact rat embryos. Sci Rep 2014;4:6382.
29. Tebas P, Stein D, Tang WW, et al. Gene editing of CCR5 in autologous CD4 T cells of persons infected with HIV. N Engl J Med 2014;370(10):901–10.
30. DiGiusto DL, Cannon PM, Holmes MC, et al. Preclinical development and qualification of ZFN-mediated CCR5 disruption in human hematopoietic stem/progenitor cells. Mol Ther Methods Clin Dev 2016;3:16067.
31. Qasim W, Zhan H, Samarasinghe S, et al. Molecular remission of infant B-ALL after infusion of universal TALEN gene-edited CAR T cells. Sci Transl Med 2017;9(374). https://doi.org/10.1126/scitranslmed.aaj2013.
32. Poirot L, Philip B, Schiffer-Mannioui C, et al. Multiplex genome-edited T-cell manufacturing platform for "off-the-shelf" adoptive T-cell immunotherapies. Cancer Res 2015;75(18):3853–64.
33. Jing W, Zhang X, Sun W, et al. CRISPR/CAS9-Mediated genome editing of miRNA-155 inhibits proinflammatory cytokine production by RAW264.7 cells. Biomed Res Int 2015;2015:326042.
34. Hacein-Bey Abina S, Gaspar HB, Blondeau J, et al. Outcomes following gene therapy in patients with severe Wiskott-Aldrich syndrome. JAMA 2015; 313(15):1550–63.
35. Kochenderfer JN, Rosenberg SA. Treating B-cell cancer with T cells expressing anti-CD19 chimeric antigen receptors. Nat Rev Clin Oncol 2013;10(5):267–76.
36. June CH, O'Connor RS, Kawalekar OU, et al. CAR T cell immunotherapy for human cancer. Science 2018;359(6382):1361–5.
37. Maude SL, Frey N, Shaw PA, et al. Chimeric antigen receptor T cells for sustained remissions in leukemia. N Engl J Med 2014;371(16):1507–17.

38. Eyquem J, Mansilla-Soto J, Giavridis T, et al. Targeting a CAR to the TRAC locus with CRISPR/Cas9 enhances tumour rejection. Nature 2017;543(7643):113–7.

39. Roth TL, Puig-Saus C, Yu R, et al. Reprogramming human T cell function and specificity with non-viral genome targeting. Nature 2018;559(7714):405–9.

40. Hoban MD, Orkin SH, Bauer DE. Genetic treatment of a molecular disorder: gene therapy approaches to sickle cell disease. Blood 2016;127(7):839–48.

41. Makani J, Ofori-Acquah SF, Nnodu O, et al. Sickle cell disease: new opportunities and challenges in Africa. ScientificWorldJournal 2013;2013:193252.

42. Huang X, Wang Y, Yan W, et al. Production of gene-corrected adult beta globin protein in human erythrocytes differentiated from patient iPSCs after genome editing of the sickle point mutation. Stem Cells 2015;33(5):1470–9.

43. Canver MC, Smith EC, Sher F, et al. BCL11A enhancer dissection by Cas9-mediated in situ saturating mutagenesis. Nature 2015;527(7577):192–7.

44. Hossain MA, Bungert J. Genome editing for sickle cell disease: a little BCL11A goes a long way. Mol Ther 2017;25(3):561–2.

45. Çiçek YA, Luther DC, Kretzmann JA, et al. Advances in CRISPR/Cas9 technology for in vivo translation. Biol Pharm Bull 2019;42(3):304–11.

46. Miller JB, Zhang S, Kos P, et al. Non-viral CRISPR/Cas gene editing in vitro and in vivo enabled by synthetic nanoparticle Co-delivery of Cas9 mRNA and sgRNA. Angew Chem Int Ed 2017;56(4):1059–63.

47. Zetsche B, Volz SE, Zhang F. A split-Cas9 architecture for inducible genome editing and transcription modulation. Nat Biotechnol 2015;33(2):139–42.

48. Zhang X-H, Tee LY, Wang X-G, et al. Off-target effects in CRISPR/Cas9-mediated genome engineering. Mol Ther Nucleic Acids 2015;4:e264.

49. Bessis N, GarciaCozar FJ, Boissier M-C. Immune responses to gene therapy vectors: influence on vector function and effector mechanisms. Gene Ther 2004;11(Suppl 1):S10–7.

50. Samulski RJ, Muzyczka N. AAV-mediated gene therapy for research and therapeutic purposes. Annu Rev Virol 2014;1(1):427–51.

51. Lee CS, Bishop ES, Zhang R, et al. Adenovirus-mediated gene delivery: potential applications for gene and cell-based therapies in the new era of personalized medicine. Genes Dis 2017;4(2):43–63.

52. Chen X, Gonçalves MAFV. Engineered viruses as genome editing devices. Mol Ther 2016;24(3):447–57.

53. Chu VT, Weber T, Wefers B, et al. Increasing the efficiency of homology-directed repair for CRISPR-Cas9-induced precise gene editing in mammalian cells. Nat Biotechnol 2015;33(5):543–8.

54. Linden RM, Ward P, Giraud C, et al. Site-specific integration by adeno-associated virus. Proc Natl Acad Sci U S A 1996;93(21):11288–94.

55. Yang Y, Wang L, Bell P, et al. A dual AAV system enables the Cas9-mediated correction of a metabolic liver disease in newborn mice. Nat Biotechnol 2016; 34(3):334–8.

56. Pack DW, Hoffman AS, Pun S, et al. Design and development of polymers for gene delivery. Nat Rev Drug Discov 2005;4(7):581–93.

57. Baum C, Kustikova O, Modlich U, et al. Mutagenesis and oncogenesis by chromosomal insertion of gene transfer vectors. Hum Gene Ther 2006;17(3):253–63.

58. Zuris JA, Thompson DB, Shu Y, et al. Cationic lipid-mediated delivery of proteins enables efficient protein-based genome editing in vitro and in vivo. Nat Biotechnol 2015;33(1):73–80.

59. Bakondi B, Lv W, Lu B, et al. In Vivo CRISPR/Cas9 gene editing corrects retinal dystrophy in the S334ter-3 rat model of autosomal dominant retinitis pigmentosa. Mol Ther 2016;24(3):556–63.
60. Latella MC, Di Salvo MT, Cocchiarella F, et al. In vivo editing of the human mutant rhodopsin gene by electroporation of plasmid-based CRISPR/Cas9 in the mouse retina. Mol Ther Nucleic Acids 2016;5(11):e389.
61. Sendra L, Herrero MJ, Aliño SF. Translational advances of hydrofection by hydrodynamic injection. Genes 2018;9(3). https://doi.org/10.3390/genes9030136.
62. Yin H, Xue W, Chen S, et al. Genome editing with Cas9 in adult mice corrects a disease mutation and phenotype. Nat Biotechnol 2014;32(6):551–3.
63. Semple SC, Akinc A, Chen J, et al. Rational design of cationic lipids for siRNA delivery. Nat Biotechnol 2010;28(2):172–6.
64. Sun Q, Kang Z, Xue L, et al. A collaborative assembly strategy for tumor-targeted siRNA delivery. J Am Chem Soc 2015;137(18):6000–10.
65. Li L, Song L, Liu X, et al. Artificial virus delivers CRISPR-Cas9 system for genome editing of cells in mice. ACS Nano 2017;11(1):95–111.
66. Lee K, Conboy M, Park HM, et al. Nanoparticle delivery of Cas9 ribonucleoprotein and donor DNA in vivo induces homology-directed DNA repair. Nat Biomed Eng 2017;1:889–901.
67. Liu J, Peng Q. Protein-gold nanoparticle interactions and their possible impact on biomedical applications. Acta Biomater 2017;55:13–27.
68. Lino CA, Harper JC, Carney JP, et al. Delivering CRISPR: a review of the challenges and approaches. Drug Deliv 2018;25(1):1234–57.
69. Ho BX, Loh SJH, Chan WK, et al. In vivo genome editing as a therapeutic approach. Int J Mol Sci 2018;19(9). https://doi.org/10.3390/ijms19092721.
70. Yu W, Wu Z. In Vivo applications of CRISPR-based genome editing in the retina. Front Cell Dev Biol 2018;6:53.
71. Li P, Kleinstiver BP, Leon MY, et al. Allele-specific CRISPR-Cas9 genome editing of the single-base P23H mutation for rhodopsin-associated dominant retinitis pigmentosa. CRISPR J 2018;1:55–64.
72. Hoffman EP, Brown RH, Kunkel LM. Dystrophin: the protein product of the Duchenne muscular dystrophy locus. Cell 1987;51(6):919–28.
73. Thanh LT, Nguyen TM, Helliwell TR, et al. Characterization of revertant muscle fibers in Duchenne muscular dystrophy, using exon-specific monoclonal antibodies against dystrophin. Am J Hum Genet 1995;56(3):725–31.
74. Tabebordbar M, Zhu K, Cheng JKW, et al. In vivo gene editing in dystrophic mouse muscle and muscle stem cells. Science 2016;351(6271):407–11.
75. Long C, Amoasii L, Mireault AA, et al. Postnatal genome editing partially restores dystrophin expression in a mouse model of muscular dystrophy. Science 2016;351(6271):400–3.
76. Nelson CE, Hakim CH, Ousterout DG, et al. In vivo genome editing improves muscle function in a mouse model of Duchenne muscular dystrophy. Science 2016;351(6271):403–7.
77. Bengtsson NE, Hall JK, Odom GL, et al. Muscle-specific CRISPR/Cas9 dystrophin gene editing ameliorates pathophysiology in a mouse model for Duchenne muscular dystrophy. Nat Commun 2017;8:14454.
78. Li D, Zhou H, Zeng X. Battling CRISPR-Cas9 off-target genome editing. Cell Biol Toxicol 2019;35(5):403–6.
79. Fu Y, Foden JA, Khayter C, et al. High-frequency off-target mutagenesis induced by CRISPR-Cas nucleases in human cells. Nat Biotechnol 2013;31(9):822–6.

80. Hsu PD, Scott DA, Weinstein JA, et al. DNA targeting specificity of RNA-guided Cas9 nucleases. Nat Biotechnol 2013;31(9):827–32.
81. Zhou H, Zhou M, Li D, et al. Whole genome analysis of CRISPR Cas9 sgRNA off-target homologies via an efficient computational algorithm. BMC Genomics 2017;18(Suppl 9):826.
82. Pattanayak V, Lin S, Guilinger JP, et al. High-throughput profiling of off-target DNA cleavage reveals RNA-programmed Cas9 nuclease specificity. Nat Biotechnol 2013;31(9):839–43.
83. Tsai SQ, Zheng Z, Nguyen NT, et al. GUIDE-seq enables genome-wide profiling of off-target cleavage by CRISPR-Cas nucleases. Nat Biotechnol 2015;33(2):187–97.
84. Kim S, Kim D, Cho SW, et al. Highly efficient RNA-guided genome editing in human cells via delivery of purified Cas9 ribonucleoproteins. Genome Res 2014;24(6):1012–9.
85. Davis KM, Pattanayak V, Thompson DB, et al. Small molecule-triggered Cas9 protein with improved genome-editing specificity. Nat Chem Biol 2015;11(5):316–8.
86. Slaymaker IM, Gao L, Zetsche B, et al. Rationally engineered Cas9 nucleases with improved specificity. Science 2016;351(6268):84–8.
87. Kleinstiver BP, Pattanayak V, Prew MS, et al. High-fidelity CRISPR-Cas9 nucleases with no detectable genome-wide off-target effects. Nature 2016;529(7587):490–5.
88. Ran FA, Hsu PD, Lin C-Y, et al. Double nicking by RNA-guided CRISPR Cas9 for enhanced genome editing specificity. Cell 2013;154(6):1380–9.
89. Cho SW, Kim S, Kim Y, et al. Analysis of off-target effects of CRISPR/Cas-derived RNA-guided endonucleases and nickases. Genome Res 2014;24(1):132–41.
90. Fu Y, Sander JD, Reyon D, et al. Improving CRISPR-Cas nuclease specificity using truncated guide RNAs. Nat Biotechnol 2014;32(3):279–84.
91. Kocak DD, Josephs EA, Bhandarkar V, et al. Increasing the specificity of CRISPR systems with engineered RNA secondary structures. Nat Biotechnol 2019;37(6):657–66.
92. Ryan DE, Taussig D, Steinfeld I, et al. Improving CRISPR-Cas specificity with chemical modifications in single-guide RNAs. Nucleic Acids Res 2018;46(2):792–803.
93. Veres A, Gosis BS, Ding Q, et al. Low incidence of off-target mutations in individual CRISPR-Cas9 and TALEN targeted human stem cell clones detected by whole-genome sequencing. Cell Stem Cell 2014;15(1):27–30.
94. Smith C, Gore A, Yan W, et al. Whole-genome sequencing analysis reveals high specificity of CRISPR/Cas9 and TALEN-based genome editing in human iPSCs. Cell Stem Cell 2014;15(1):12–3.
95. Scott DA, Zhang F. Implications of human genetic variation in CRISPR-based therapeutic genome editing. Nat Med 2017;23(9):1095–101.
96. Tsai SQ, Topkar VV, Joung JK, et al. Open-source guideseq software for analysis of GUIDE-seq data. Nat Biotechnol 2016;34(5):483.
97. Lazzarotto CR, Nguyen NT, Tang X, et al. Defining CRISPR-Cas9 genome-wide nuclease activities with CIRCLE-seq. Nat Protoc 2018;13(11):2615–42.
98. Tsai SQ, Nguyen NT, Malagon-Lopez J, et al. CIRCLE-seq: a highly sensitive in vitro screen for genome-wide CRISPR-Cas9 nuclease off-targets. Nat Methods 2017;14(6):607–14.
99. Wienert B, Wyman SK, Richardson CD, et al. Unbiased detection of CRISPR off-targets in vivo using DISCOVER-Seq. Science 2019;364(6437):286–9.

100. Lamarche BJ, Orazio NI, Weitzman MD. The MRN complex in double-strand break repair and telomere maintenance. FEBS Lett 2010;584(17):3682–95.
101. Kosicki M, Tomberg K, Bradley A. Repair of double-strand breaks induced by CRISPR-Cas9 leads to large deletions and complex rearrangements. Nat Biotechnol 2018;36(8):765–71.
102. Akcakaya P, Bobbin ML, Guo JA, et al. In vivo CRISPR editing with no detectable genome-wide off-target mutations. Nature 2018;561(7723):416–9.
103. Kim J, Hu C, Moufawad El Achkar C, et al. Patient-customized oligonucleotide therapy for a rare genetic disease. N Engl J Med 2019;381(17):1644–52.
104. Aiello C, Terracciano A, Simonati A, et al. Mutations in MFSD8/CLN7 are a frequent cause of variant-late infantile neuronal ceroid lipofuscinosis. Hum Mutat 2009;30(3):E530–40.
105. Finkel RS, Chiriboga CA, Vajsar J, et al. Treatment of infantile-onset spinal muscular atrophy with nusinersen: a phase 2, open-label, dose-escalation study. Lancet 2016;388(10063):3017–26.
106. Research C for DE and. Expanded access to investigational drugs for treatment use - questions and answers. U.S. Food and Drug Administration. 2019. Available at: http://www.fda.gov/regulatory-information/search-fda-guidance-documents/expanded-access-investigational-drugs-treatment-use-questions-and-answers. Accessed November 29, 2019.
107. Research C for BE and. Expedited programs for regenerative medicine therapies for serious conditions. U.S. Food and Drug Administration. 2019. Available at: http://www.fda.gov/regulatory-information/search-fda-guidance-documents/expedited-programs-regenerative-medicine-therapies-serious-conditions. Accessed November 29, 2019.
108. Research C for BE and. Regulatory considerations for human cells, tissues, and cellular and tissue-based products: minimal manipulation and homologous use. U.S. Food and Drug Administration. 2019. Available at: http://www.fda.gov/regulatory-information/search-fda-guidance-documents/regulatory-considerations-human-cells-tissues-and-cellular-and-tissue-based-products-minimal. Accessed November 29, 2019.

The Future of Clinical Diagnosis

Moving Functional Genomics Approaches to the Bedside

Rini Pauly, MS*, Charles E. Schwartz, PhD

KEYWORDS

- Whole-genome sequencing (WGS) • RNA sequencing
- Genome wide methylation/Epi-signatures • Functional assay • Metabolomics
- Proteomics • Multi-omic analysis

KEY POINTS

- Whole-genome sequencing (WGS) identifies critical alterations in the genome that are not present in the coding genes.
- Genome-wide methylation studies identify epi-signatures that allow clarification and proper classification of variants of uncertain significance.
- RNA-seq, both targeted and untargeted, allows diagnosis of human disorders, particularly those in patients with a suspicious phenotype and no obvious genomic alteration.
- Bioinformatics tools, and neural networks, allow for the association of apparently unrelated events.
- Multi-omic analysis—the integrated analysis of data from various omic studies (WGS, methylation, RNAseq)—identifies coordinated interaction of variants leading to a phenotype.

INTRODUCTION

Sequencing techniques are limited by the interpretation of a large number of coding and noncoding, sequence and structural, variants. In-silico tools for predicting the impact of coding variants and regulatory elements have become increasingly advanced. However, the evidence from these tools is generally not sufficient for accurate variant classification. In this article, the authors discuss a multi-omic approach that they foresee will enable genome-wide characterization and classification of

This article originally appeared in *Advances in Molecular Pathology*, Volume 2, 2019.
Greenwood Genetic Center, JC Self Research Institute, 113 Gregor Mendel Circle, Greenwood, SC 29646, USA
* Corresponding author.
E-mail address: rpauly@ggc.org

variants by integrating several omics data, assisted by bioinformatics tools and deep learning algorithms for variant prioritization. These prioritizations can then be quantified using advanced high-throughput functional assays.

SIGNIFICANCE

Interpreting the clinical impact of variants of uncertain significance (VUSs) and eventually the joint effect of having multiple variants in the same or different genes is complex. A multi-omic approach promises to address this compound issue of variant assessment by combining genomic, transcriptomic, epigenomic, and functional proteomic data using novel computational tools. Accumulation and accessibility of these data will eventually lead to a comprehensive variant effect map, a significant step toward accurate clinical interpretation of genetic variants.

CURRENT CLINICAL VARIANT INTERPRETATION APPROACHES

Rapid advances in genomic technologies is changing the traditional practice of medicine to primarily include predictive, preventive, and personalized medicine approaches.[1,2] However, the central challenge for clinical genomics remains in conclusive interpretation of the numerous novel variants found through DNA sequencing. Increasingly, sequencing-based technologies in research and clinical laboratories are detecting large number of variants for which the clinical significance is unknown. Such variants are also called variants of uncertain significance (VUSs). In 2015, the American College of Medical Genetics and Genomics and the Association for Molecular Pathology[3] published standards and guidelines for sequence variant interpretation and to ensure accurate and consistent variant classification. This guideline outlines the evidence used in variant classification including population, computational, functional, segregation and allelic data, and conservation analyses among other variant evidence. Different pieces of evidence are weighed differently (supporting, moderate, strong, very strong) and then combined to reach a final classification (pathogenic, likely pathogenic, VUSs, likely benign, benign) for any given variant.

Often times, there is not enough clinical or functional evidence to support variant classification leading to an assimilation of a large number of VUSs. Therefore, there is a need for additional testing modalities across laboratories to improve the reproducibility and objectivity of variant interpretation. These might include primarily genomic, epigenetic, transcriptomic, proteomic, and metabolomic modalities. Data from all such modalities may then be combined and analyzed, using high-throughput computational systems, to determine the clinical significance of the relevant genetic variant (**Fig. 1**).

WHOLE-GENOME SEQUENCING

The implementation of genomic medicine in the clinic has long being recognized as an essential component in providing good clinical care. Although exome sequencing is cost and time efficient, it focuses on only ~1% to 2% of the genome, unlike whole-genome sequencing (WGS) that covers 95% to 98% of the genome. WGS has several advantages when compared with exome and targeted panels including uniform coverage in coding and noncoding regions, which allows detection of copy number variants (CNVs) and structural variants. Specifically, WGS has demonstrated the use of paired-end sequencing to obtain breakpoint resolution of CNVs, rearrangements, and other structural variations.[4–7] Several medical centers and commercial laboratories across the United States have now implemented genome sequencing programs

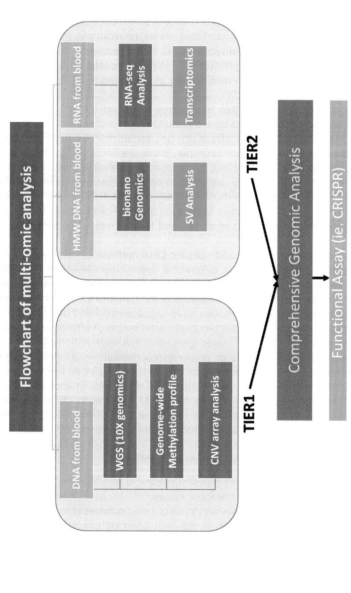

Fig. 1. Steps for human multi-omic analysis that combines multiple technologies to identify and characterize non-linear relationships between variants and genes in a single disorder or several related disorders. WGS; Whole-genome sequencing, CNV; Copy number variants, HMV; High Molecular Weight, bionano genomics; non-sequencing-based genome mapping technology to identify structural variants and create de novo genome assemblies, SV; Structural Variant, CRISPR; Clustered Regularly Interspaced Short Palindromic Repeats.

with "in-house" sequencing and analysis of variants with review and sign-out by a board-certified clinical molecular geneticist. However, the pace of the clinical application of WGS has been limited due to various factors including cost, insurance coverage, and data storage limitations.

EPIGENOMICS AND PREDICTION OF VARIANTS IMPACT

Epigenetic changes, through DNA methylation and histone modifications, can modulate gene expression and the overall cellular and/or systems phenotype.[8–10] There are several ways to obtain enriched methylated sequences, for example, methylated DNA immunoprecipitation-sequencing, methylated CpG island recovery assay, or whole-genome shotgun bisulfite sequencing (WGBS).[11,12] WGBS, considered the "gold standard", enables the detection of DNA methylation at single base-pair resolution. The treatment of DNA with sodium bisulfite allows the discrimination of methylated and unmethylated cytosines. However, this technology is limited by the DNA quantity and quality that can be compromised by the desulfonation process.

Furthermore, the epigenetic modifications can be used as markers for molecular diagnostics and disease screening. For example, there are 3 commercially available DNA methylation-based diagnostic tests for colorectal cancer: EpiproColon, Colo-Vantage, and RealTime mS9 that are designed to detect hypermethylated SEPT9 in a blood sample. EpiproColon is the most clinically validated diagnostic epigenetic biomarker for colon cancer. Noninvasive tests such as these are preferred over colonoscopy by patients, thereby serving as an efficient tool for molecular screening and diagnosis.[13]

Schenkel and colleagues[14] developed specific DNA methylation signature assays for Fragile X syndrome by identifying differential methylation levels at the FMR1 gene promoter. Separately, Choufani and colleagues[15] used the same approach to identify additional aberrant methylation loci across the genome for Sotos syndrome. Recently, syndrome-specific epi-signatures were characterized and used to support the classification of VUSs and the unambiguous identification of affected individuals. In 2018, Aref-Eshghiand colleagues[16] used genomic DNA methylation signatures to support the classification of variants in neurodevelopmental syndromes, including 14 Mendelian disorders. This novel approach was further developed to characterize overlapping peripheral blood DNA methylation epi-signatures in individuals with Coffin-Siris and Nicolaides Baraitser syndromes.[17] More recently, this application was expanded to include 19 conditions[18] and became the first epigenetic signature test (EpiSign) for inherited disorders in the United States and Europe.[19]

RNA-SEQ ANALYSIS AND PREDICTION OF VARIANTS IMPACT

RNA-seq is increasingly being seen as a powerful clinical tool to improve diagnostic yield in genetically unresolved and complex cases.[20,21] In 2017, Kremer and colleagues[22] investigated the utility of RNA-seq in diagnosing patients with mitochondrial disorders. The study identified several genes with aberrant expression, abnormal splicing events, and/or allele-specific expression (mono-allelic expression), whereby one allele is silenced, leaving only the other allele expressed. These findings lead to the molecular diagnosis of 5 out of 48 undiagnosed patients with mitochondriopathies along with and identification of candidate genes to establish novel disease-gene association in other cases. In another publication, Cummings and colleagues[23] explored RNA-seq as a complementary diagnostic tool to genomic sequencing by systematically detecting transcript level changes, mainly aberrant splicing events. The added diagnostic yield of RNA-seq in this study was 35%. Using this approach, a highly recurrent, disruptive intronic variant was identified in the *COL6A1* gene in a total of 27 genetically unsolved collagen VI-like dystrophy patients. Overall, both these studies demonstrated the power of RNA-seq for detection and classification of variants missed by standard genomic diagnostic approaches.

Gonorazky and colleagues[24] developed PAGE (Panel Analysis of Gene Expression), a web-based tool to promote RNA sequencing-based diagnostics for rare Mendelian diseases. PAGE supports the comparison of gene expression across multiple tissues and identification of variants and splicing changes through this analysis. This study focused on monogenetic neuromuscular disorders as proof of principle to provide genetic resolution in 36% (9/25) of cases. Their diagnostic algorithm compared 70 undiagnosed individuals with an in-house database and with control transcriptome data obtained from the Genotype-Tissue Expression (GTEx) project. GTEx is a database of 53 nondisease tissue sites across nearly 1000 individuals. It includes tissue-specific gene expression data (RNA-seq) combined with WGS or WES data.[25] This transcriptome database catalogs many naturally occurring genetic variants that modulate alternative splicing and consequently influence phenotypic variability and disease susceptibility in human populations.

APPLICATION OF VARIANT FUNCTIONAL ASSAYS IN METABOLOMICS

Metabolomics is the comprehensive analysis of metabolites within a biological system and can be a valuable tool in deciphering the clinical significance of VUSs. Chong and colleagues[26] developed an open source tool, MetaboAnalyst, which facilitates integrative analysis to identify biologically meaningful patterns in quantitative metabolomic data. Such tools are valuable in rapidly classifying multiple patterns in complex datasets. In 2013, Boccuto and colleagues[27] used phenotype microarrays for metabolic profiling of lymphoblastoid cells from 137 patients with neurodevelopmental disorders with or without autism spectrum disorders (ASDs) and 78 normal individuals. Phenotype MicroArray assays are mammalian cell-based assays used to investigate up to 1400 metabolites in mammalian cells in a high-throughput manner. Using this system, the investigators identified decreased tryptophan metabolism as a potential unifying biochemical basis for patients with ASDs, which could be pursued further as a first diagnostic assay for ASDs. This platform also allows the characterization of the metabolic profile of ASD cells, which will then help in understanding the impact of rare novel variants on ASD genes. Another neurologic disorder, Snyder-Robinson syndrome, was first reported in 1969[28] as an X-linked intellectual disability syndrome and until very recently was the only known genetic disorder associated with the polyamine metabolic pathway. Li and colleagues[29] successfully uncovered some of the mechanisms underlying the pathologic consequences of abnormal polyamine metabolism in the nervous system by identifying a distinctive shift in the metabolism of carbon energy sources that further indicates a compromised mitochondrial function. This is another example where such a specific metabolic signature can be used to characterize VUSs associated with this disease.

HIGH-THROUGHPUT FUNCTIONAL ASSAYS AND DEEP LEARNING MODELS

In 2018, Findlay and colleagues[30] developed a saturation genome editing assay to characterize 96.5% of all possible single-nucleotide variants (SNVs) in 13 (out of 24) exons of the *BRCA1* gene. This region is known to play a key role in the tumor suppressor function. This assay was designed using the CRISPR/Cas9 approach to alter each nucleotide for a total of about 4000 possible individual mutations. The frequency of the induced variant was used to score its effect on *BRCA1* function. It was found that the functional effects were concordant with assessments of pathogenicity from ClinVar. This included more than 400 missense SNVs, as well as around 300 SNVs that disrupt expression. This approach can be extended to overcome the challenge of VUSs in additional clinically actionable genes.

Separately, Starita and colleagues[31] also developed and published a multiplex Homology-directed DNA Repair Assay to measure the effects of more than 1000 *BRCA1* missense substitutions on DNA repair in breast and ovarian cancer. They were able to demonstrate an accurate discrimination of loss-of-function versus benign missense variants with 87.5% sensitivity and 100% specificity.

Taking a different approach, Drost and colleagues,[32] in 2018, developed a Cell-free *In vitro Mismatch Repair Activity* (CIMRA) assay to enhance the classification of VUSs in the DNA mismatch repair genes in Lynch syndrome. Their CIMRA assay allows generation and functional analysis of several variants of the MLH1 protein in vitro at the same time. The investigators tested 26 *MLH1* variants and of these, 15 had lost activity. Further, these results match up with the in silico and pathology data. High-throughput functional assays such as this will enable fast and accurate classification of VUSs; however, their clinical implementation still requires more work to address feasibility, clinical validity, and infrastructure requirements.

A well-validated functional assay could ultimately be used as a clinical annotation tool to study the impact of the variant on a protein's function, its effect on cellular function, and its ability to be used as a drug target.[33] The major bottleneck for functional studies is that most VUSs are rare (ie, seen in one or very few patients) but are collectively numerous. Therefore, fast, cost-effective and high-throughput functional assays are needed to assess the effect of a large number of possible variants in any given gene or molecular pathway. Three benchmark studies in 2010 to 2011 by Fowler and colleagues,[34] Ernst and colleagues,[35] and Hietpas and colleagues[36] led to the development of deep mutational scanning. These studies initiated the use of multiplexed assays for variant effect (MAVEs) that could create comprehensive atlas of functional data for 10^4–10^6 variants in a single experiment. The multiplexed assays accomplished this by linking the genotype of each variant to its effect in a functional assay.[37] Different MAVE approaches have been established, but they share a common process. Variants are synthesized, introduced into a model system, and carefully chosen for a phenotype of interest.

Massively parallel reporter assays use a library of mutagenized promoter sequences, to calculate the effect of a promoter variant on expression by using the read ratio of RNA-seq to DNA-seq data.[38,39] Researchers at the University of Alabama at Birmingham (UAB) developed a blood-based functional RNA assay for the *NF1* (*neurofibromin 1*) gene, which enabled identification of 2.5% (>65 different locations harboring deep intronic splice variants) of all known pathogenic deep intronic splice variants in the *NF1*UAB cohort.[40–42]

Recently, Evans and colleagues[43] used clinical sequencing data from more than 17,000 patients to train a disease-specific variant pathogenicity predictor that approached 100% accuracy for several epilepsy, cardiomyopathy, and RASopathies genes. Another deep neural network application predicts the clinical impact of a human mutation using primate species. Unlike previous efforts that lacked adequately sized datasets containing confidently labeled benign and pathogenic variants for training, Sundaram and colleagues[44] demonstrated that common missense variants in other primate species are largely clinically benign in human, enabling pathogenic mutations to be systematically identified by the process of elimination. Using thousands of common variants from population sequencing of 6 nonhuman primate species, they trained a deep neural network that identifies pathogenic mutations in patients with rare disease with 88% accuracy and enabled the discovery of 14 new candidate genes in intellectual disability genome wide. This kind of comprehensive cataloging of common variation from additional primate species would advance genome variant interpretation and further improve the clinical utility of human genome sequencing.

MULTI-OMIC ANALYSIS

The technologies mentioned in this article have the potential to improve the characterization of molecular phenotypes in normal and disease tissues by capturing of genomic, epigenomic, and transcriptomic profiles. However, an integrated analysis of these heterogeneous data sets to diagnose diseases is not straight forward and is still not within the capacity of most clinical laboratories. Argelaguet and colleagues[45] introduced MOFA, a framework for unsupervised integration of multi-omics data sets in chronic lymphocytic leukemia (CLL) and mouse embryonic stem cells. MOFA was done in 2 steps. In step 1, data were collected from 200 patients to assess single-cell RNA expression and DNA methylation and their response to drugs. In step 2, the single-cell expression and methylation data were used to identify coordinated transcriptional and epigenetic changes along cell differentiation. This application accurately detected mislabeled samples and imputed missing values but most importantly was able to identify major sources of disease heterogeneity in CLL, that is, somatic mutation status of the immunoglobulin heavy-chain variable region gene and chromosome 12 trisomy status. Another study by Singh and colleagues,[46–48] used a factor model integrative approach for identifying key molecular drivers from multiomic assays. Data Integration Analysis for Biomarker discovery using Latent Components identifies both known and novel multi-omics biomarkers consisting of mRNAs, miRNAs, CpGs, proteins, and metabolites. Although most studies integrate omics data for testing marginal associations between different data types, they still lack an overall interpretability. A major limitation of this approach is relying on a linear model, which means that it would not detect nonlinear relationships between the input features. The authors propose a multi-omics strategy that aims to go from genotype to phenotype.

However, in order for this approach to attain its full potential, one needs an interactive omics platform to fully understand the choreography of genes, cells, tissues, organs, and environment.[1] The platform should enable building and implementation of computational analytical tools to be able to identify nonlinear relationships between variants and genes and across different datasets.

Although a comprehensive omic analysis platform is set in place, advanced functional assays are still needed to quantify these findings. For instance, CRISPR could be applied to create multiple single edits in a control cell line to recapitulate the original patient profile.[48] The advantages of this technique is that it allows in situ modification, which can be done at a genome-wide scale for specific sites of interest and it can be used in the proper cell type using iPS cell technology. This platform would certainly serve as an accomplished start for clinical reporting and personalized genomic medicine.

SUMMARY

Recent years have seen an exponential increase in VUS findings. A large number of missense variant entries in ClinVar are classified as VUSs.[33] Although there have been some commendable coordinated efforts to produce, analyze, and share these large complex datasets, we are long way from addressing the variant interpretation challenge. In order to progress, we need to recognize intermediate steps that lie between genomic discovery research and evidence-based clinical implementation.

Comprehensive variant assessment programs need to be implemented to assess a variant's impact on protein function and to integrate multiple lines of evidence to expedite efficient variant classification, providing improved benefit for patients.[49,50] In addition, it will become necessary to undertake what we term human multi-omic analysis to solve disorders resulting from a single variant or from the interaction of multiple variants. Finally, using high-throughput functional assays will be a powerful tool for VUS classification in Mendelian and complex disorders.

ACKNOWLEDGMENT

This work is supported in part by a grant from the South Carolina Department of Disabilities and Special Needs (SCDDSN).

REFERENCES

1. Green ED, Guyer MS. Charting a course for genomic medicine from base pairs to bedside. Nature 2011;470(7333):204–13.
2. MuzafarBeigh M. Next-generation sequencing: the translational medicine approach from "bench to bedside to population" (vol. 3). Medicines 2016;3(2):14.
3. Richards S, Aziz N, Bale S, et al. Standards and guidelines for the interpretation of sequence variants: a joint consensus recommendation of the American College of Medical Genetics and Genomics and the Association for Molecular Pathology. Genet Med 2015;17(5):405–24.
4. Stavropoulos DJ, Merico D, Jobling R, et al. Whole genome sequencing expands diagnostic utility and improves clinical management in pediatric medicine. NPJ Genom Med 2016;1:15012.
5. Caspar SM, Dubacher N, Kopps AM, et al. Clinical sequencing: from raw data to diagnosis with lifetime value. Clin Genet 2018;93(3):508–19.
6. Mostovoy Y, Levy-Sakin M, Lam J, et al. A hybrid approach for de novo human genome sequence assembly and phasing. Nat Methods 2016;13:587.
7. Barseghyan H, Tang W, Wang RT, et al. Next-generation mapping: a novel approach for detection of pathogenic structural variants with a potential utility in clinical diagnosis. Genome Med 2017;9(1):90.
8. Egger G, Liang G, Aparicio A, et al. Epigenetics in human disease and prospects for epigenetic therapy. Nature 2004;429(6990):457–63.
9. Gibney ER, Nolan CM. Epigenetics and gene expression. Heredity 2010;105:4.
10. Lim DH, Maher ER. DNA methylation: a form of epigenetic control of gene expression. Obstet Gynaecol 2010;12:37–42.
11. Li D, Zhang B, Xing X, et al. Combining MeDIP-seq and MRE-seq to investigate genome-wide CpG methylation. Methods 2015;72:29–40.
12. Li Y, Tollefsbol TO. DNA methylation detection: bisulfite genomic sequencing analysis. MethodsMol Biol 2011;791:11–21.
13. Issa IA, Noureddine M. Colorectal cancer screening: an updated review of the available options. World J Gastroenterol 2017;23(28):5086–96.
14. Schenkel LC, Schwartz C, Skinner C, et al. Clinical validation of fragile X syndrome screening by DNA methylation array. J Mol Diagn 2016;18(6):834–41.
15. Choufani S, Cytrynbaum C, Chung BHY, et al. NSD1 mutations generate a genome-wide DNA methylation signature. Nat Commun 2015;6:10207.

16. Aref-Eshghi E, Rodenhiser DI, Schenkel LC, et al. Genomic DNA methylation signatures enable concurrent diagnosis and clinical genetic variant classification in neurodevelopmental syndromes. Am J Hum Genet 2018;102(1):156–74.
17. Aref-Eshghi E, Bend EG, Hood RL, et al. BAFopathies' DNA methylation episignatures demonstrate diagnostic utility and functional continuum of Coffin–Siris and Nicolaides–Baraitser syndromes. Nat Commun 2018;9(1):4885.
18. Aref-Eshghi E, Bend EG, Colaiacovo S, et al. Diagnostic utility of genome-wide DNA methylation testing in genetically unsolved individuals with suspected hereditary conditions. Am J Hum Genet 2019. https://doi.org/10.1016/j.ajhg.2019.03.008.
19. Genome web, April 2019. Available at: https://www.genomeweb.com/molecular-diagnostics/first-epigenetic-signature-test-inherited-disorders-launch-us-europe. Accessed July 22, 2019.
20. Li D, Tian L, Hakonarson H. Increasing diagnostic yield by RNA-Sequencing in rare disease-bypass hurdles of interpreting intronic or splice-altering variants. Ann Transl Med 2018;6(7):126.
21. Byron SA, Van Keuren-Jensen KR, Engelthaler DM, et al. Translating RNA sequencing into clinical diagnostics: opportunities and challenges. Nat Rev Genet 2016;17:257.
22. Kremer LS, Bader DM, Mertes C, et al. Genetic diagnosis of Mendelian disorders via RNA sequencing. Nat Commun 2017;8:15824.
23. Cummings BB, Marshall JL, Tukiainen T, et al. Improving genetic diagnosis in Mendelian disease with transcriptome sequencing. Sci Transl Med 2017;9(386) [pii:eaal5209].
24. Gonorazky HD, Naumenko S, Ramani AK, et al. Expanding the boundaries of RNA sequencing as a diagnostic tool for rare mendelian disease. Am J Hum Genet 2019;104(3):466–83.
25. GTEx portal. Available at: https://gtexportal.org/home/. Accessed July 22, 2019.
26. Chong J, Soufan O, Caraus I, et al. MetaboAnalyst 4.0: towards more transparent and integrative metabolomics analysis. Nucleic Acids Res 2018;46(W1): W486–94.
27. Boccuto L, Chen C-F, Pittman AR, et al. Decreased tryptophan metabolism in patients with autism spectrum disorders. Mol Autism 2013;4(1):16.
28. Lauren Cason A, Ikeguchi Y, Skinner C, et al. X-linked spermine synthase gene (SMS) defect: the first polyamine deficiency syndrome. Eur J Hum Genet 2003; 11:937.
29. Li C, Brazill JM, Liu S, et al. Spermine synthase deficiency causes lysosomal dysfunction and oxidative stress in models of Snyder-Robinson syndrome. Nat Commun 2017;8(1):1257.
30. Findlay GM, Daza RM, Martin B, et al. Accurate classification of BRCA1 variants with saturation genome editing. Nature 2018;562(7726):217–22.
31. Starita LM, Islam MM, Banerjee T, et al. A multiplex homology-directed DNA repair assay reveals the impact of more than 1,000 BRCA1missense substitution variants on protein function. Am J Hum Genet 2018;103(4):498–508.
32. Drost M, Tiersma Y, Thompson BA, et al. A functional assay–based procedure to classify mismatch repair gene variants in Lynch syndrome. Genet Med 2018. https://doi.org/10.1038/s41436-018-0372-2.
33. Starita LM, Ahituv N, Dunham MJ, et al. Variant Interpretation: Functional Assays to the Rescue. Am J Hum Genet 2017;101(3):315–25.
34. Fowler DM, Araya CL, Fleishman SJ, et al. High-resolution mapping of protein sequence-function relationships. Nat Methods 2010;7(9):741–6.

35. Ernst A, Gfeller D, Kan Z, et al. Coevolution of PDZ domain-ligand interactions analyzed by high-throughput phage display and deep sequencing. MolBiosyst 2010;6(10):1782–90.
36. Hietpas RT, Jensen JD, Bolon DNA. Experimental illumination of a fitness landscape. Proc Natl Acad Sci U S A 2011;108(19):7896–901.
37. Weile J, Roth FP. Multiplexed assays of variant effects contribute to a growing genotype-phenotype atlas. Hum Genet 2018;137(9):665–78.
38. Movva R, Greenside P, Marinov GK, et al. Deciphering regulatory DNA sequences and noncoding genetic variants using neural network models of massively parallel reporter assays. PLoS One 2019;14(6):e0218073.
39. Hoskinson DC, Dubuc AM, Mason-Suares H. The current state of clinical interpretation of sequence variants. CurrOpin Genet Dev 2017;42:33–9.
40. Koczkowska M, Chen Y, Callens T, et al. Genotype-phenotype correlation in NF1: evidence for a more severe phenotype associated with missense mutations affecting NF1codons 844–848. Am J Hum Genet 2018;102(1):69–87.
41. RNA-based NF1testing on blood: Available at: https://www.uab.edu/medicine/genetics/medical-genomics-laboratory/testing-services/nf1-legius-syndrome-and-rasopathies/nf1-via-rna. Accessed July 22, 2019.
42. Zhou J, Theesfeld CL, Yao K, et al. Deep learning sequence-based ab initio prediction of variant effects on expression and disease risk. Nat Genet 2018;50(8):1171–9.
43. Evans P, Wu C, Lindy A, et al. Genetic variant pathogenicity prediction trained using disease-specific clinical sequencing data sets. Genome Res 2019 Jul;29(7):1144–51.
44. Sundaram L, Gao H, Padigepati SR, et al. Predicting the clinical impact of human mutation with deep neural networks. Nat Genet 2018;50(8):1161–70.
45. Argelaguet R, Velten B, Arnol D, et al. Multi-omics factor analysis-a framework for unsupervised integration of multi-omics data sets. Mol Syst Biol 2018;14(6):e8124.
46. Singh A, Shannon CP, Gautier B, et al. DIABLO: an integrative approach for identifying key molecular drivers from multi-omics assays. Bioinformatics 2019. https://doi.org/10.1093/bioinformatics/bty1054.
47. Ipe J, Swart M, Burgess KS, et al. High-throughput assays to assess the functional impact of genetic variants: a road towards genomic-driven medicine. ClinTranslSci 2017;10(2):67–77.
48. Perrino C, Barabási AL, Condorelli G, et al. Epigenomic and transcriptomic approaches in the post-genomic era: path to novel targets for diagnosis and therapy of the ischaemic heart? Position Paper of the European Society of Cardiology Working Group on Cellular Biology of the Heart. Cardiovasc Res 2017;113(7):725–36.
49. Zhu Y, Tazearslan C, Suh Y. Challenges and progress in interpretation of noncoding genetic variants associated with human disease. ExpBiol Med (Maywood) 2017;242(13):1325–34.
50. Woods NT, Baskin R, Golubeva V, et al. Functional assays provide a robust tool for the clinical annotation of genetic variants of uncertain significance. NPJ Genom Med 2016;1:16001.

Printed and bound by CPI Group (UK) Ltd, Croydon, CR0 4YY

03/10/2024

01040481-0011